Enhancing Treatment Benefits with Exercise

Enhancing Treatment Benefits with Exercise

Interventions for Mood, Anxiety, Cognition, and Resilience

WORKBOOK

MICHAEL W. OTTO
JASPER A. J. SMITS

OXFORD
UNIVERSITY PRESS

OXFORD
UNIVERSITY PRESS

Oxford University Press is a department of the University of Oxford. It furthers
the University's objective of excellence in research, scholarship, and education
by publishing worldwide. Oxford is a registered trade mark of Oxford University
Press in the UK and certain other countries.

Published in the United States of America by Oxford University Press
198 Madison Avenue, New York, NY 10016, United States of America.

© Oxford University Press 2024

All rights reserved. No part of this publication may be reproduced, stored in
a retrieval system, or transmitted, in any form or by any means, without the
prior permission in writing of Oxford University Press, or as expressly permitted
by law, by license, or under terms agreed with the appropriate reproduction
rights organization. Inquiries concerning reproduction outside the scope of the
above should be sent to the Rights Department, Oxford University Press, at the
address above.

You must not circulate this work in any other form
and you must impose this same condition on any acquirer.

CIP data is on file at the Library of Congress

ISBN 978–0–19–094899–3

DOI: 10.1093/med-psych/9780190948993.001.0001

Printed by Marquis Book Printing, Canada

MWO: To Whitney, the real athlete in the family, you truly shine in every way

JAJS: To Jill and Stella, for many happy exercise sessions

One of the most difficult problems confronting patients with various disorders and diseases is finding the best help available. Everyone is aware of friends or family who have sought treatment from a seemingly reputable practitioner, only to find out later from another doctor that the original diagnosis was wrong or the treatments recommended were inappropriate or perhaps even harmful. Most patients, or family members, address this problem by reading everything they can about their symptoms, seeking out information on the internet or aggressively "asking around" to tap knowledge from friends and acquaintances. Governments and health-care policymakers are also aware that people in need do not always get the best treatments—something they refer to as *variability in health-care practices.*

Now health-care systems around the world are attempting to correct this variability by introducing *evidence-based practice.* This simply means that it is in everyone's interest that patients get the most up-to-date and effective care for a particular problem. Health-care policymakers have also recognized that it is very useful to give consumers of health care as much information as possible, so that they can make intelligent decisions in a collaborative effort to improve physical health and mental health. This series, Treatments *ThatWork*™, is designed to accomplish just that. Only the latest and most effective interventions for particular problems are described, in user-friendly language. To be included in this series, each treatment program must pass the highest standards of evidence available, as determined by a scientific advisory board. Thus, when individuals suffering from these problems or their family members seek out an expert clinician who is familiar with these interventions and decides that they are appropriate, patients will have confidence they are receiving the best care available. Of course, only your health-care professional can decide on the right mix of treatments for you.

Many clinicians emphasize the importance of mind/body integration for achieving overall health and well-being. There can be no better example of this philosophy than the use of exercise to improve mental health. And it works! There is substantial evidence that exercise can be used to treat depression, anxiety, and panic; enhance cognition; reduce stress; and enhance psychological resilience. Given these benefits, exercise can also be targeted to specific problem areas such as aiding smoking cessation. Quite simply, readers will be surprised by the scope of benefits exercise can offer to mental health. Your clinician may have referred you to this exercise program as a stand-alone treatment, as an addition to other ongoing treatment, or as a strategy to extend gains or prevent relapse following success with a prior treatment. Regardless of the reason, there is no wrong time to start an exercise for mental health program.

The motivational strategies in this workbook offer you a fresh way to approach exercise and make the program work for your lifestyle. In addition to information on how to start and maintain and exercise program, this workbook comes complete with worksheets and logs for scheduling and tracking your physical activity. Exercise-based treatment offers what you need, and the guidance provided by this workbook helps you get to and stay with a successful exercise program to enjoy a better mood, less anxiety, better cognition, and a general sense of psychological resilience.

David H. Barlow, Editor-in-Chief,
Treatments *That Work*™
Boston, MA

Contents

Michael W. Otto, PhD, is Professor in the Department of Psychological and Brain Sciences and Director of the Translational Research Laboratory at Boston University. He has had a major career focus on developing and validating new psychosocial treatments, with a focus on treatment-refractory populations including those with mood, anxiety, and substance use disorders. His work includes a translational research agenda investigating brain–behavior relationships in therapeutic learning. Dr. Otto's focus on hard-to-treat conditions and principles underlying behavior-change failures led him to an additional focus on health-behavior promotion, including investigations of addictive behaviors, medication adherence, sleep, and exercise. Dr. Otto has published over 480 articles and 20 books spanning his research interests, and he was identified as a "top producer" in the clinical empirical literature as well as an ISI Highly Cited Researcher. He received the APA Society of Clinical Psychology award for Distinguished Scientific Contributions to Clinical Psychology, the Elizabeth Hurlock Beckman Award from the American Psychological Association for Mentoring, and the Toy Caldwell-Colbert Award for Distinguished Educator in Clinical Psychology. His leadership positions include serving as President of the Association of Behavioral and Cognitive Therapies, and President of Division 12 of the American Psychological Association.

Jasper A. J. Smits, PhD, is Professor of Psychology and Director of the Anxiety & Health Behaviors Laboratory at the University of Texas at Austin. He specializes in the development and evaluation of behavioral interventions for anxiety and related disorders. With respect to exercise, he has been involved in research testing whether aerobic training can provide learning experiences (e.g., feeling safe around bodily sensations, reappraisal of stressors) essential to attaining patients' treatment goals. Following up on initial successes in this area among adults with anxiety motivated to quit smoking, he has developed a YMCA exercise-based smoking cessation intervention that is currently undergoing evaluation. Dr. Smits has authored over 250 publications, frequently provides workshops on exercise for mental health, and maintains an active private practice.

GOALS

- To learn about this treatment program
- To identify the symptoms and goals you want to address
- To select your support team
- To work with your therapist and physician to decide on your level of activity

OVERVIEW

This workbook is designed to help you structure and maintain an exercise program to improve your mood, anxiety, cognition, resilience, or habit control (smoking). The use of exercise for these mental health targets is supported by a wealth of research evidence. It is clear from large-scale surveys that individuals who exercise have less stress, less anxiety, less depression, better cognition (e.g., better memory and attention), and fewer substance use problems than those who don't exercise. For example, studies show that a program of exercise can be used to treat depression and can achieve results that rival those provided by antidepressant medication or psychotherapy. Likewise, programmed exercise has been found to be useful for the management of anxiety problems, including the treatment of panic disorder. There is also an abundance of evidence that exercise can be used to address some of the cognitive impairments that can occur with aging as well as specific disease processes like Alzheimer's disease or

Parkinson's disease. Finally, because exercise promotes resilience in general, and aids mood management and tolerance of symptoms, exercise can help individuals quit smoking (or help with other habits where low mood or intolerance of symptoms leads to relapse). For whatever treatment goals you choose, this workbook will provide you with information about using exercise to target mental health challenges.

We recommend that you begin this program by reading and working through Chapters 1 through 4, which discuss common issues and solutions relevant for planning an exercise program. Starting, maintaining, and supplementing your exercise program is the focus of Chapters 5 through 7. Then we provide chapters devoted to specific symptoms. Using your exercise program to treat depression is covered in Chapter 8, with additional information on bipolar disorder in Chapter 9. Anxiety disorders are the focus of Chapter 10. Chapter 11 provides information on exercise to enhance cognition. Chapter 12 focuses on the general goal of enhancing psychological resilience, and Chapter 13 discusses the use of exercise to help stop smoking or other habits. The final chapter (Chapter 14) discusses additional strategies for maintaining an exercise program over the long term. One copy of each worksheet is included at the end of the chapter where the worksheet is introduced, and additional copies can be accessed (and downloaded) by searching for this book's title on the Oxford Academic platform, at academic.oup.com.

Why a Formal Treatment Program for Exercise?

You probably already know that regular exercise is good for your mood and good for your body. Nonetheless, it can be hard to start or maintain an exercise program, particularly when feeling depressed or anxious. This workbook is structured to help you adopt skills to create a regular exercise program as well as prevent mood disturbances from blocking the very activities that can help you feel better.

We assume that during this program, you will encounter multiple barriers to exercise, especially including the ways in which a low mood or over-busy schedule will sap your motivation to get out and exercise. For this reason, this workbook gives you tips to make it easier to start the habit of regular exercise. This workbook also offers ways of thinking about, scheduling, and monitoring your exercise program to help you keep motivated by making it easier to start exercising and easier to notice the benefits of exercising.

But I Have Been *Trying* to Exercise!

Exercising for specific mental health benefits is very different from exercising for general health benefits. When you exercise for general health, you have to work *now* to get general health benefits *later*. And when you feel sad, stressed, or anxious, it is very hard to do something in the present for the purpose of a future health benefit. However, if the goal of exercising is to stop feeling bad *now*, it becomes much easier to follow through with exercise despite having a negative mood. Over time, exercise can become the activity that you do because you want a mood lift. The fact that you also get in good shape and better your physical health is just an extra benefit. This program asks you to exercise to feel good, and because of this, feeling bad is never a reason to skip exercise. Feeling bad now *is* the very reason to exercise now!

Why Start an Exercise Program?

One of the first things you will do in this program is clarify your motivations for starting an exercise program. Exercise should be a personally rewarding activity for you. Using Worksheet 1.1: Symptoms to Be Targeted by Exercise, review and identify some of the symptoms you want to address with your exercise program. Worksheets can be found at the end of this chapter or can be accessed by searching for this book's title on the Oxford Academic platform, at academic.oup.com.

As mentioned, exercise also has a wide variety of benefits other than mental health benefits. We want you to be aware of these benefits, and using Worksheet 1.2: Other Benefits of Exercising, check off those you care more about.

Again, this program doesn't ask you to exercise just because of these longer-term health benefits. It wants you to exercise to feel good *now*—to improve your mood, have less anxiety, have a better memory, and have better control over habits that hurt your health. Nonetheless, know that when you exercise for these mental health reasons, not only are you likely to feel better, you are also likely to have better overall health and a longer lifespan.

Thinking About Your Support Team

Because exercise may be a new habit for you, you will want to have a support team. Using Worksheet 1.3: Selecting Members of Your Support Team, consider who you might want to encourage you or participate with you in your new exercise program. Take a few moments to think about who will be most supportive of your goal to develop an exercise habit. Then, consider how exercise might change your social life. Are there people with whom you would like to exercise, or are there additional social activities that you might pursue because you will be in better shape? Select members of your support team and, using the worksheet, list them in the space provided. Remember, worksheets can be found at the end of this chapter or can be accessed by searching for this book's title on the Oxford Academic platform, at academic.oup.com.

Also, keep in mind that your general levels of energy and comfort when engaging in activities may increase as you achieve your exercise goals. Chapter 7 has you consider additional pleasant activities that may support you in this new lifestyle. That is, regular exercise may lead to new interests in pickleball, or swimming, or joining the local volleyball team. With greater fitness you will find that you may have removed barriers that kept you from other enjoyable activities.

Working with Your Therapist

This workbook is designed for use in conjunction with a program of exercise supervised by a therapist (a psychologist, physician, nurse, social worker, or mental health counselor). Your therapist should play an active role in deciding if this exercise program is right for you. Some therapists will recommend exercise after you have tried medications or psychotherapy as a way to manage your mood, anxiety, cognition, or habits. Others will recommend exercise as a first step in helping you manage your mood. Regardless of the timing of this exercise intervention, know that you have a wide variety of choices in getting help for your mood, anxiety, or stress levels. No single treatment works for everyone.

Cognitive-behavioral therapy, general psychotherapy, medications, or stress management programs can all provide benefits. As a good consumer, consider these options along with exercise as is needed for you to reach your mood and anxiety management goals or your cognitive or habit control goals.

Knowing Your Physical Limitations

We commonly recommend that you undergo a full medical evaluation with your physician before starting an exercise program. It is important to know your current level of physical health and to be aware of any physical conditions that should limit your participation in exercise. Let your physician know that you are about to start an exercise program that is targeting the public health–recommended dose for adults from the American College of Sports Medicine and the American Heart Association. Depending on your level of fitness, you may work up to this level slowly. In addition, please make sure to have a detailed discussion with your physician if you have problems with chest pain, breathing difficulties, light-headedness, bone or joint pain, or high blood pressure, or if you are taking medications for a heart condition or high blood pressure. Even with these conditions, this exercise program might be right for you, but the decision about your level of activity should be made in consultation with your physician.

Breaking Free of the Past

Before you go on to the next chapters in this workbook and learn more about how exercise can help with a broad range of mental health goals, and before you start to consider what sort of exercise program you want to pursue, we would like you to pause and look back at your history of exercise. Some people who are starting this program are lapsed athletes; they were active for years and defined themselves in part by their physical abilities. Other people coming to this program were never regular exercisers, and in fact may have been reluctant to ever join in with individual or team sports. Some people coming to this program loved the shape of their body; others did not. Some liked being in the pool, some hated being on the track, and some swore never to play a ball sport again.

Regardless of your own history with exercise, we would like you to come to an exercise-for-mental-health program with fresh expectations. We don't want you to remember how fast or slow you were when you had to run laps in gym class. We don't care whether you were picked first or last for the kickball game, and we really don't think it matters whether you picked up extra pounds in the last year or two. We want you to come to this exercise program as you are now. We want you to see if there are ways to make exercise more fun than it used to be. And we want to make sure that you use exercise for its mental health benefits. In the chapters that follow, we will give you some specific information about exercise characteristics you may want to consider, but at every point we want you to find out what sort of exercise fits into your lifestyle now, and if possible, find out how you can use exercise to fit with other relaxation-time, social-time, or recreation-time goals.

Please check off the mood symptoms you would like to work on.

Symptoms of Depression

_______________ Sad or blue mood

_______________ Loss of interest in things you care about

_______________ Feelings of guilt about things done or not done

_______________ Low energy and difficulties being motivated to start or finish activities

_______________ Poor concentration

_______________ Disrupted appetite or loss of interest in eating

_______________ Feelings of agitation or lethargy

_______________ Feelings that nothing matters

_______________ Difficulties sleeping or poor sleep quality (or oversleeping)

Symptoms of Anxiety

_______________ General anxiety

_______________ Worry

_______________ Feelings of anticipation

_______________ Feeling jumpy

_______________ Startling easily

_______________ Panic attacks

_______________ Avoidance of situations (write in situations:)

_______________ Poor concentration

_______________ Problems with sleep

_______________ Feeling tense

_______________ General feelings of stress

Cognitive Symptoms

_______________ Difficulties with memory

_______________ Difficulties concentrating

_______________ Having a harder time following directions

_______________ Trouble focusing your attention for longer tasks

_______________ Worries about a family history of dementia

Habit Control (Smoking)

_______________ Difficulties staying on track with goals when frustrated or anxious

_______________ Feeling pushed around by craving or withdrawal sensations

_______________ A desire to cut down or quit smoking or vaping

_______________ Failures to stay off cigarettes due to low mood

Other Symptoms You Want to Work on

____

____

____

Worksheet 1.2: Other Benefits of Exercising

Frequent exercise can help you to:

____ Manage weight

____ Lower cholesterol

____ Lower hypertension

____ Prolong lifespan

____ Enhance strength and endurance

____ Reduce risk of heart disease

____ Enhance immune functioning

____ Improve sleep

____ Reduce fatigue

_______________________________________ Make it easier to complete physical activities

___________________Find new hobbies that require greater physical fitness than I have now

Who would be happy that you are exercising and might encourage you in this program?

____

____

____

Who might you select for support because they have an important impact on your life?

____

____

____

Who might you want to have join you in your new exercise habit—by being with these people during exercise or seeing them after exercise?

____

____

____

CHAPTER 2

How Exercise Works for Your Mental Health Goals

GOALS

- To learn about how exercise works to help mood, anxiety, cognition, and resilience (specific intervention strategies for these topics are detailed in workbook Chapters 8–13)
- To understand the importance of moderation
- To recognize the limitations of exercise in managing mood
- To consider other treatment options as warranted

OVERVIEW

There is now a wealth of evidence that exercise is a useful treatment for low mood and depression, with increasing evidence for similar benefits for anxiety disorders and resilience for habit control. Exercise is also one of the best treatments available today to improve cognition and protect brain function. The following pages present some of the current perspectives on why exercise has these beneficial effects. Knowing how exercise works when it comes to improving your mental health can help you pay attention to these aspects of your exercise program.

Research on biological changes associated with regular exercise has shown that exercise leads to changes in some of the same neurotransmitters (chemicals in our brains) targeted by antidepressant medications used to treat both mood and anxiety disorders. The broad action of exercise for both of these conditions is consistent with the broad action of these medications. One way in which exercise may work is by stimulating the brain chemical serotonin. Serotonin is an important neurotransmitter for the regulation of emotion and is the main neurotransmitter affected by medication such as Paxil®, Prozac®, Zoloft®, and Celexa®. These medications modify the activity of neurons sensitive to serotonin; likewise, regular exercise appears to have effects on serotonin activity. And there are broader actions as well. In addition to modifying serotonin functioning, there is evidence that exercise can also change other aspects of brain functioning, including changes to brain regions dependent on the neurotransmitter noradrenaline and the functioning of the neurotransmitter GABA; GABA functioning is a central target of many antianxiety drugs like the benzodiazepines (e.g., Xanax®, Ativan®).

The Importance of the Memory Molecule BDNF for Cognition

Exercise also has important effects on a crucial brain-maintenance molecule known as BDNF (brain-derived neurotrophic factor). BDNF has been called a memory molecule because it is involved in the way the brain forms memories, helping these memories to be available for guiding ongoing functioning. In addition, BDNF also has broader functions helping your brain neurons grow and thrive. These two functions of BDNF—directly aiding shorter- and longer-term memory and supporting your brain's functioning overall—are two reasons why your therapist may have used a Miracle-Gro® metaphor in describing the benefits of exercise for cognition. Just like Miracle-Gro ®can support the growth and thriving of plants, BDNF has similar functions for the brain. Importantly, each bout of exercise is metaphorically similar to pouring Miracle-Gro® over the brain. And, when you are more fit, more metaphorical Miracle-Gro® is poured over the brain with each bout of exercise. These actions are thought to be the primary reason why exercise enhances attention and memory as well as helping treat the loss of brain functioning with aging and from specific brain diseases like Alzheimer's disease.

One of the specific benefits of exercise is increased tolerance of the physical and emotional symptoms of anxiety. Being better able to tolerate anxiety-related sensations (such as a rapid heart rate, trembling, or feeling breathless) is an important feature of resilience. With increased comfort with sensations of anxiety, people are less likely to avoid anxiety-provoking situations. Imagine what it would be like to sit through an important meeting, naturally feeling anxious but less bothered by that anxiety so that you can better focus on the meeting and your goals. This is a benefit of exercise, particularly if you and your therapist work to pay attention to and enhance these benefits.

Chapter 10 describes the importance of becoming more comfortable with anxiety sensations for the treatment of anxiety and panic disorder. Likewise, Chapter 12 in this workbook describes the importance of becoming comfortable with the natural experience of anxiety for enhancing resilience, and Chapter 13 discusses the application of this sort of resilience for coping with mood, anxiety, and withdrawal symptoms that are part of the process of quitting smoking. A common theme across these chapters is using exercise to become more comfortable with a range of uncomfortable bodily sensations, so that those sensations cannot "push you around." By "push you around" we mean the ways in which trying to escape or avoid uncomfortable bodily sensations like those encountered when you are anxious can have powerful effects in limiting your lifestyle by encouraging avoidance. There is strong evidence that regular exercise can help people become more comfortable with bodily sensations regardless of their source, and can also help people become more comfortable with their own experience of anxiety. This means that individuals can use exercise as a general tool to help them to be less pushed around by the sensations they experience. When you become more comfortable with your own experience of anxiety, it will be easier for you to choose how to react to anxiety sensations, rather than feeling like anxiety is choosing your actions for you.

Stress and Sleep Management

In addition to more direct effects on neurotransmitters involved in mood, exercise may also have indirect effects on mood by helping to normalize sleep patterns. Sleep problems can be related to both mood and anxiety disorders. Medication treatments for these conditions often improve sleep, and likewise there is evidence that exercise can improve sleep. Since sleep normalization is important to support your exercise habits and mood, Chapter 7 provides additional discussion of good sleep habits.

The period following your bout of exercise may also be important for achieving broader mood benefits from exercise. The feelings of relaxation, well-being, and accomplishment that can follow a successful exercise episode may be significant in further calming anxiety and easing depression. During this time, a person may be less likely to be affected by some of the negative thinking patterns of depression, making it easier to view the next several hours after exercise in a more positive light. Even a few hours of relief from the overwhelming feelings of depression or anxiety may work like a crowbar to give leverage for moving away the full syndrome of these disorders. For this reason, try to be particularly mindful of the benefits of exercise in the hours after a bout of exercise. This will help enhance your desire to exercise on the following day, and such mindfulness may also play an important role in driving away negative moods.

Also, the beneficial effects of exercise on reducing feelings of stress may have importance for *preventing* both mood and anxiety disorders. Stressful events challenge mood, and in a number of studies, stress has been linked to relapse in depressive or anxiety disorders. To the extent that exercise can help you manage feelings of stress, it can help you prevent the onset or relapse of these disorders.

Activity Levels

As will be discussed in Chapters 8 through 10, many of the disorders that exercise can help have self-perpetuating cycles that involve low activity or avoidance. Exercise may work in part because it returns the body to helpful action and can increase your resilience to negative mood states, regardless of whether your goal is to push through feeling bad, or to get involved in more activities, or to better tolerate the blues that can happen when trying to quit smoking. As you learn to exercise independently of the way you feel, the meaning of your negative emotions might change. Sad or anxious feelings may start to feel less overwhelming, and as you stay active despite low moods, these episodes of low mood should lessen.

It is important to keep a balance of exercise and rest, with attention to giving your body the moderation it needs to promote mood stability. We talk about this in Chapter 9, which discusses using exercise to help with bipolar disorder. The direct antidepressant effects of exercise, along with normalizing your sleep, balancing the sleep–wake cycle, and achieving a balanced schedule of activity, may be helpful in calming some of the depressed moods and unstable moods that are at the heart of bipolar disorder. Also, because some of the pharmacological treatments for bipolar disorder have the side effect of weight gain, the effects of regular exercise on weight control may be an additional appealing aspect of this program for individuals with bipolar disorder.

What Exercise Does Not Treat

Using exercise to help manage mood and anxiety disorders does *not* mean you should ignore other treatment options. There is ample evidence that certain types of psychotherapy and medication are effective for treating mood and anxiety disorders. Exercise can be considered as a complement to these approaches or can be tried on its own. If you don't achieve the results you desire with this program, we strongly recommend seeking consultation to consider other treatment approaches. And, at every point, it is important for you to be a good consumer of treatment options.

Using exercise to dampen stress is not a substitute for the use of good problem-solving skills. Likewise, using exercise to change how you react to emotions is not a substitute for fuller examination of emotional patterns in your life. For example, along with using exercise to reduce the effects of stress, you may need to plan how to better manage the stressors in your life. Aim to always strike a balance between considering what your body needs and using the body to calm the mind, while also making sure that you use all the resources you can to aid your mood management. This is especially true if you have serious worsening of symptoms or ever have suicidal thoughts. Suicidal thoughts are a symptom of depression, and it is important that you treat such thoughts as a symptom *in need of immediate treatment*. Any thoughts of self-injury should be discussed with a qualified clinician.

Your mind and body are connected, and in this exercise program, you are intervening with the body to help the mind and mood. As such, exercise is an especially fitting partner to psychotherapy. To balance the focus in psychotherapy on talking, understanding, feeling, and planning, exercise helps keep you focused on doing, moving, and achieving. Exercise will help you establish healthy patterns of activity and rest, with a balance of each.

This workbook aims to help you provide treatment to yourself—to give yourself what your body needs to help your mind and emotions stay in balance. As part of being an informed consumer, you can get more information on the nature and treatment of mood and anxiety disorders from the National Institute of Mental Health on the Web site at www.nimh. nih.gov/health/topics/.

GOALS

- To learn how to motivate yourself by taking steps *toward* exercise
- To choose a time to exercise in your daily schedule
- To plan for exercise (clothes, music, route, etc.)
- To research online and local resources (optional)
- To find an exercise partner or group (optional)

OVERVIEW

Starting a new program of regular exercise is challenging. Everyday life events, hassles, and bad habits can interfere with our best intentions. The good news is that many of these obstacles are predictable, understandable, and avoidable. In this chapter, you will be introduced to some of the situational factors that can interfere with establishing a program of regular exercise. Also, you will start becoming familiar with how to tackle these patterns and how to create situations to help support your exercise goals.

Motivation

A useful starting point in thinking about barriers to exercise is to consider the concept of MOTIVATION. We often think of motivation as a stable inward trait that precedes behavior change and helps us to determine the success of our goals and intentions—but this is not necessarily true. A strong motivation to change does not always *precede* useful behavior change. This is because the desire to do something often *follows* the successful completion of the behavior. It is by doing something one or more times that we can establish the inward desire (the motivation) to do it again. As such, at the start of this program, we do not expect you to have a strong feeling that exercise is important. That feeling may well come *after* you have successfully changed your mood, anxiety, or stress through exercise.

Changing Conditions to Enhance Motivation

Because motivation can follow rather than precede useful habits, it is important to make new habits easy enough to start and maintain rather than just hope for motivation. Also, feelings of motivation are richly dependent on the external environment as well as your current thoughts and mood. The key is to make changes in your environment in order to enhance your motivation. In short, rather than simply expecting yourself to feel like exercising, this program will have you *arrange the conditions* so you will more naturally feel like exercising.

Consider the following situation. When coming home from work, and finally getting a chance to sit down and relax, it can be overwhelming to think about getting back up and completing a workout. From the vantage point of sitting on the couch, getting up and going to the gym is really hard. The key is not to overwhelm yourself with such hard expectations. All you need to do is put yourself in the condition where going to the gym or doing some form of exercise is a more natural thought. So, instead of focusing on getting yourself to exercise, *focus only on the next step* that will make it more likely that you will exercise.

From the position of being on the couch, the first goal is helping yourself take one step toward being ready for exercise, such as putting on your exercise clothes. Once you have your workout clothes on, you become a different person of sorts. Instead of being "couch person" who can only feel like staying on the couch, you become "workout person" for whom taking the next steps toward exercise feels like the right answer. You may not feel like stepping outside to run, but you might feel like doing a couple warm-up exercises. And doing those warm-up exercises can make you feel more like stepping outside for a run or grabbing your keys to go to the gym. The key is not to tell yourself that you should go to the gym, but to consider what small things you could do to help you feel like an "exerciser" so that you more naturally want to work out.

A few helpful reminders about the payoff of exercise may also help—perhaps a note in your left running shoe that says "mood" to remind yourself of one of the many benefits of working out. And speaking of those shoes, keep them handy. Having to look too long for a missing shoe is a great way to derail motivation for a workout. Figure 3.1 illustrates this process of chaining together some small steps to get yourself to your workout.

Using Example 3.1: Exercise Stuck Points, think about situations where you might "get stuck" trying to get yourself to exercise. Record them in the space provided. For many people, the topmost difficult situation might be television time, where it is easy to think, "Let me just sit here for a while longer."

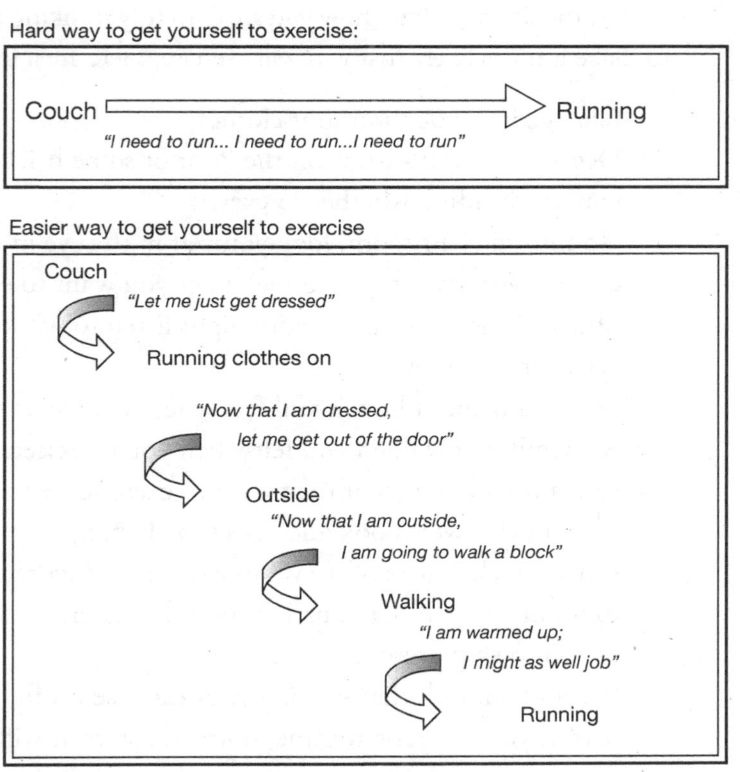

Figure 3.1

Setting the Stage for Exercise Success

Exercise 3.1: Exercise Stuck Points

Think about situations where you might get stuck trying to get yourself to exercise and write these down on the lines below.

____

____

____

____

____

After completing Exercise 3.1, try to identify a few things that might help you get off the couch and exercise. Remember that the only goal is to have you change the situation (and how you are currently thinking and feeling) enough to make it more likely that you will exercise. Here are a few suggestions:

- Change into your workout clothes.
- Decide to do 10 sit-ups on the floor or some brief stretching while you are deciding whether to exercise.
- Go into the bathroom, look yourself in the eye in the mirror, and discuss with your reflection whether you want to exercise..
- Think of the good music you might listen to while exercising and go get your music player.
- Daydream about how it will feel when you are done exercising.
- Remember how good you felt when you exercised last.
- Call a friend and see if they want to exercise.
- Get out this workbook and review a chapter.
- Get yourself a glass of ice water to prepare (hydrate) for exercise.
- Remind yourself that a bad mood is a reason to exercise, not a reason to skip exercise.
- Remind yourself that starting your exercise is often the most difficult part of your exercise routine; once you start, it will get easier.

Then using Exercise 3.2: Changing Situations to Change Motivation for Exercise, write your own ideas in the space provided.

Exercise 3.2: Changing Situations to Change Motivation for Exercise

Identify a few things that might help you shift your motivation by shifting the situation you are in. The goal is to find small ways to move yourself off the couch and toward exercise. Write your ideas down on the lines below.

____

____

____

____

____

Making It Easier to Exercise: Timing

To avoid exercise feeling like a battle of motivations, consider ways of setting up your exercise schedule so that it will fit your lifestyle and maximize your urge to exercise. The following sections are designed to help you think about some of the factors that can be important in the process of making it easier to exercise, starting with the timing of your exercise.

When it comes to supporting a new exercise habit, first think through some of the things that may make it easier to start and keep doing your exercise program. That is, the timing of when you plan to exercise can make a big difference for how well you complete it. If possible, schedule exercise around natural breaks in your day and for when it is likely to make you feel best. Also, because exercise typically involves a change of clothes and, in many cases, a shower afterwards, it is important to plan how these disruptions fall into your daily routine.

Morning Exercise

Some individuals select morning exercise as a way to start the day. Advantages of an early workout include:

- Exercise is an excellent way to start the day.
- The exercise shower becomes the morning daily shower.
- Morning time may allow better weather conditions.

- Early morning time is excellent "me time."
- All day you get to enjoy the sense of accomplishment of having already exercised.

Challenges to morning exercise include *difficulties getting out of bed for exercise*. Because most people are limited on time because of work, school, or home demands in the morning, delays in getting out of bed can seriously interfere with morning exercise time. Also, early in the morning—when you are only half-awake—it is difficult to make decisions. Make the decision about whether you are going to exercise before going to bed. Then stick to this decision. Be careful of motivation-sapping thoughts such as the following:

- *I will skip my workout just this one time.*
- *It is too cold to get out of bed.*
- *It will be more valuable for my mood if I sleep in.*
- *Missing my workout once won't matter.*

Beware of delaying tactics that close out or substantially reduce your exercise time. Remember that you made your decision to exercise when you had an *awake mind* the previous evening. Don't let any of the following thoughts have the power to push you away from exercising (and these thoughts do have lots of power for a half-awake mind):

- *I will just turn over in bed one more time before I get up.*
- *Staying in bed 10 more minutes won't matter.*
- *I am too tired to exercise well.*
- *I can always exercise this evening.*

Anticipating your reactions the night before you are scheduled to exercise may help you counter your arguments against starting exercise the next morning. Having these thoughts hit you in the morning may then even bring a smile to your face and motivate you to get started.

Afternoon Exercise

An afternoon exercise break is an excellent way to manage stress. It can make use of a segmented day (e.g., the long lunch and break before a return to work that is so popular in European countries). With a fixed midday break for exercise, the workday can lose its marathon quality. There is the morning work routine, and then a break in which the levels of stress are reduced. During this break, the body gets to be active and the mind gets to rest. Then, one can return to the afternoon physically tired but mentally refreshed and ready to meet home, work, school, or personal goals. One of the major challenges to getting out for the midday exercise break is the tendency to *one more thing* yourself away from having time to exercise. Thoughts characterizing this "one more thing" tendency include the following:

- *I am working well; I will get just one more thing done.*
- *I am too busy. I better not take a break till later.*
- *If I don't finish this now, it will be too overwhelming later.*

To counter these motivation-sapping thoughts, you will need to remind yourself that exercise may enhance your problem-solving levels while reducing your stress. You may be physically tired after exercise, but your productivity may shoot up due to having a clear and refreshed mind. So to counter the above "one more thing" thoughts, you may want to remind yourself that:

- *I am taking a break to exercise to have a fresh mind for my afternoon job demands.*
- *I know that I feel different after exercise; let me see what work feels like under those conditions.*
- *I have a mountain of housework, but that will be easier to face once I get a workout in.*
- *Management of my stress and mood is one way I am helping myself be more productive.*

Evening Exercise

Evening exercise can be a terrific way to close out the day and prepare for an especially relaxed and enjoyable evening. Some people use evening exercise as a way to close out the workday and reduce stress prior to being with family or friends. Others may be able to incorporate a run into their commute home or use exercise and the post-exercise shower and change of clothes as their way to prepare for an enjoyable evening. The change in focus brought by exercise and a post-exercise shower can be useful for enhancing your interpersonal interactions. For example, it can help you shift your attention to the joys that can be found at home or in your social life rather than hurrying off and bringing the day's residue of work with you.

Exercising approximately 3 hours before sleep is also a good way to give yourself time to recover from exercise and take advantage of some of the natural sedating properties of a good workout.

One of the challenges of evening exercise is that you may need to cope with exercise avoidance due to fatigue from the day. Motivation-sapping thoughts about working out in the evening include:

- *I am too tired. I can just put it off until morning.*
- *It is about to get dark.*
- *It will be too cold.*

To help you resist such thoughts, be careful with how you manage your surroundings. If you go home and sit on the couch, the likelihood that you will get back up and exercise is greatly reduced. Consider how you can exercise right after work or school. Alternatively, see if you can integrate exercise into the family routine. Jogging strollers are a terrific tool for the busy parent who wants to exercise. The child in the stroller may be lulled to sleep or may entertain you with conversation while you walk, jog, or run.

Combining Motivations the "Exercise+" Way

There is no reason to depend on the joy of exercise alone to help keep you motivated for your new exercise program. Whenever possible we would like you to combine motivations, so that your exercise time is "Exercise+ ." We have already mentioned the use of music or audiobooks to enhance your exercise experience, but there are lots of additional strategies for you to consider. In each case, you are looking for something that you like to do (is motivating) that you are going to add to your exercise. The goal is to make your exercise time feel more special by combining it with something else you enjoy so that you will feel an added pull toward exercising. Consider the following examples.

- Exercise+ can provide you with time to just relax and listen to your audiobook (playing the audiobook exclusively when you are on a walk).
- Exercise+ can represent an opportunity to unwind before getting home from work (setting up a regular exercise session at the gym as part of your commute home).

- Exercise+ can help you keep in touch with your old friend from work now that you have changed jobs (arranging a weekly doubles tennis game).
- Exercise+ can involve getting to meet a new group of people (attending meet-up runs organized by your local sports store).

In setting up an Exercise + program for yourself, think about what sort of activities or events you are currently missing out on (*"I don't have enough time to read fiction;" "I don't get to see my friend John much anymore"*). Then consider how these activities might be combined with exercise. Some of these considerations may change how you choose to exercise. For example, you may choose pickleball over running so you can meet with John regularly. Or you may choose to regularly ride a recumbent bike at the gym so you can move through several seasons of *Breaking Bad* or *Bridgerton* on your smartphone and still get your workouts done.

An Exercise+ program does take some motivation, and there are a few ground rules. If you are listening to a podcast for your Exercise+, listen to it *only* when exercising (keeping your headphone jack tied to the handle of your workout bag might be a good reminder). If you are using meetings with John to help you play tennis, don't let yourself switch to meeting at a bar for beer instead. You want to keep a strong (and exclusive) link between exercise and the + so that wanting the + naturally pulls you into your exercise.

Planning Your Exercise

Besides timing, there are several other factors to consider in planning your exercise.

Clothes and Music

Wearing comfortable clothes and dressing appropriately for the weather (with care toward protecting against being too hot or too cold) can make a big difference in your enjoyment of exercise. Also, because exercise can heat the body so well, you may find that you have to layer your clothes, perhaps taking off a jacket and tying it around your waist after you complete the initial minutes of exercise.

Also, exercising with music can greatly increase the joy of exercise. For example, the authors of this workbook are deeply committed to running while listening to music, podcasts, or audiobooks. Running in time to a song or losing oneself in an engaging book is an excellent way to enhance enjoyment while exercising. However, some care needs to be taken when wearing headphones to avoid dangerous situations; sounds of passing cars, bikes, dogs, and rollerbladers can be blocked by loud music or narration on headphones. Be sure to take extra care (e.g., exercising with just one earphone in place) when exercising in busy areas.

The selection of exercise clothes and exercise music can form a pleasant reward for good exercise habits. Many of the clothes available in sport stores have amazing properties to allow air exchange and wick away moisture, while also providing protection from the cold. Investment in clothes that make you feel good can help support your exercise habit. Likewise, investment in good headphones and a way to carry your sound device (clips, handhelds, etc.) can help make exercise more pleasurable.

Planning Your Route

Running, jogging, or walking is a particularly accessible exercise that requires no equipment (other than appropriate shoes); because of this we use running/jogging/walking as a frequent way to encourage new exercisers. You may choose a different exercise, but we will nonetheless use running, jogging, or walking to illustrate some of the principles for organizing your exercise in this and following chapters. Especially early on in your exercise training program, planning your running/jogging/walking route beforehand may help you mentally prepare for your exercise session. Consider using distance markers (e.g., a specific intersection, post office, or school) to help you break up your activity into smaller parts that are each linked to a feeling state (e.g., hard, smooth, struggle, and easy). For example, that first section from your house to the traffic light may always be the most challenging part of your run—you are still a bit stiff and your muscles may feel tight. However, once you get to the traffic light, you have warmed up and hitting the pavement feels much better. Anticipating a difficult beginning that has an end and will be followed by a segment during which you feel much better will likely increase your motivation to get started. The authors of this workbook frequently use the free mapping service offered by MapMyRun (http://www.mapmyrun.com) to plan their running activities.

You may also want to engage in some exercise tourism. If you haven't gotten to visit local parks in your area, or that new walking space down by the river (for example), you may want to plan your exercise around getting to see new sites and getting to know new neighborhoods. If you are deciding to walk rather than run, you might also consider how you can integrate your walking with doing errands. Bring a backpack and get that errand to the drugstore out of the way with a couple-mile walk. But always consider your surroundings: Not all neighborhoods are safe for walking and running, and not all neighborhoods have sidewalks. Choose your routes well for your longer-term health and safety.

Tracking Your Heart Rate

If you like devices and are curious about how hard you are working during your exercise, you may want to consider purchasing a heart rate monitor. These simple-to-use and relatively cheap devices help you to track the fluctuation in your heart rate during exercise, which will guide you in setting and modifying intensity. These devices also allow you to estimate your average exercise-session heart rate, which will help you determine whether you are receiving the recommended exercise dose (see Chapter 5).

Exercise Partners

Exercise partners can be invaluable in helping you keep up a regular exercise schedule. Knowing that you are not alone in a new habit is always helpful, and having someone ask about your routine and your achievements can provide a useful motivational boost. In addition, for any joint exercise plans (meeting a partner for tennis, meeting a friend for a walk), the social pressure provided by having another person counting on you to show up for a workout can be a powerful tool for keeping you on track.

Refer to your completed Worksheet 1.3: Selecting Members of Your Support Team, at the end of Chapter 1 of this workbook, to consider who might be a good exercise partner. This partner does not have to accompany you on all of your workouts; even a weekly partner can provide the extra support and change-up from your regular patterns to help establish an interesting and fun exercise habit.

Other Support Systems

A number of local clubs or programs may be available to support your exercise habit. For example, USA FIT is a commercial exercise support network that may be available in your city. USA FIT helps people prepare to complete exercise goals (e.g., completing a half-marathon) by providing them with a training program complete with coaching, moral support, and connections to others with similar training goals. Fitlink and MapMyRun are other services that provide connections to others, including information on workouts and motivational issues experienced by others. They also give users the ability to create personal profiles online, track workout results, and search for exercise partners. These services share in common a web-based approach to helping you network with and feel more connected to others in your exercise efforts. Because the quality and nature of services on the internet can change over time, be a good consumer and check the following and other links with an eye toward making sure the services are right for you:

- USA FIT: http://www.usafit.com
- Fitlink: http://www.fitlinkapp.com
- MapMyRun: http://www.mapmyrun.com.

Other resources that may be available in your area include running clubs, walking clubs, biking clubs, and, of course, workout gyms. Local sporting goods stores are often a good resource for identifying clubs in your area. Drop by the store and ask the salesperson about groups that may be available in your area. It can't be overestimated how much easier it is to exercise when you have people expecting you to exercise with them.

GOALS

- To observe your thoughts and redirect them as needed
- To practice helpful thinking strategies *during* exercise
- To practice helpful thinking strategies *after* exercise
- To practice helpful thinking strategies *hours after* exercise

OVERVIEW

One powerful tool you have in helping yourself keep up with your exercise habit is to actively manage your thinking patterns. Thoughts can have a powerful effect on influencing mood and can either boost or sap motivation. In Chapters 8 through 10, we provide specific attention to the role of negative thoughts in mood and anxiety disorders. This chapter provides strategies for thinking about exercise in a useful way.

Enjoying the Present

So much of our thinking is future- or past-oriented: How has the day/week/month gone so far? What needs to be done next hour? What needs to be done next week? With all this thinking, it is often hard to realize what is going on *in the moment* or to be engaged enough in the moment to enjoy it. Exercise will naturally help you bring your attention back to the moment, but we want to make sure that you are ready to enjoy this effect. Indeed, one useful feature of exercise is that it is difficult to keep on worrying or having repeated negative thoughts in your head (ruminating) while you are exercising. Exercise can help you develop the "quiet mind" that is at the heart of many meditative techniques. Rather than thinking, monitoring, reviewing, and rehashing, the goal is to simply *experience* the current moment. To become better at experiencing, though, it is helpful to become better at noticing your current thinking habits.

Observing Your Thoughts

In preparation for getting the most out of exercise-related changes in cognitions (such as memory and paying attention), it will be important to become a good observer of the tone and content of your thoughts. To help you learn about your thinking patterns, pick a regular event that you can use as a signal for you to observe your own thinking. It can be any regularly occurring event, like the ringing of an hourly wristwatch chime, each time you open the front door to leave the house, or each time you open the refrigerator to start preparing a snack or meal. You can use these events to remind you to stop and notice whether your thoughts are present-, past-, or future-oriented.

Remembering to Check Your Thoughts

One of the authors' favorite cues for observing thoughts is sitting at a stoplight—when waiting for a red light to change, examine ("listen in on") your thoughts. Ask yourself, "What am I thinking about right now? Where am I directing my mental energies?"

At a red light, you have the opportunity to do any number of pleasant activities: actively listen to the radio, hum a tune, daydream about a recent pleasant event, or plan an enjoyable event or interaction for the evening. If you find you are doing one of those things, good for you. But many readers will find they are doing none of these things; they are instead ruminating about problems—potential problems, past problems, future problems, nonexistent problems—or focusing on the traffic or on the stoplight itself ("Why won't you change!"). None of these topics add pleasure to your life, yet you may discover this is where you are devoting your mental energies.

Redirecting Your Thoughts

Try to use stoplights as your chance to start changing these patterns. When at a stoplight, notice where your thoughts go, observe the effect they have on you (how they make you feel), and then, if they are not contributing to your well-being in the moment, redirect them to a more pleasurable or useful topic. You may even want to continue to think about a problem, but make sure that it is active problem-solving, not just thinking about the negative aspects of a situation. With regular stoplight practice (and practice with your wristwatch chime, front door, refrigerator door, etc.), you will have a better sense of where your thoughts tend to go and more experience with gently redirecting them. Remember, the task is to:

1. Notice your thoughts.
2. Observe how these thoughts make you feel.
3. Redirect the thoughts to a more useful or pleasurable topic.

By learning about the nature of thinking, and becoming better at observing and redirecting thoughts, you will be more prepared to make use of your exercise program. That is, you will be better able to take advantage of exercise's effect of decreasing constant negative thoughts and avoiding some of the bad habits that can sap some of the joy of exercise.

Thinking Strategies During Exercise

The ultimate goal for exercise is to have your thoughts centered on the present and, if possible, on the most pleasurable aspects of your exercise session. If running outside, for example, this will include noticing the look of nature (sky, trees, color of grass, shadings of snow), interesting sights and surroundings (other people, buildings), pleasant daydreams, or the sound of music or an audiobook. If running inside, you may need to focus on daydreaming, music, or the sights and sounds of the gym.

Redirecting Negative Thoughts

In contrast to paying attention to the pleasurable aspects of running and your surroundings, it is sometimes easy to become focused on negative thoughts about running, which seem to recur with every step:

- *When will I be done? When will I be done? When will I be done?*
- *I don't like this. I don't like this. I don't like this.*

If you find yourself engaged in these bad habits, gently redirect your thinking, using gentle coaching with thoughts such as:

- *Ooh. This sort of thinking and attention isn't helping me. What else can I daydream about that might be more fun?*
- *"When will I be done?" Let me focus on what is interesting during the run. Let me take a good look at the view.*
- *I have not been listening to my music. How can thinking about being done be more interesting than this song? Let me refocus my efforts and feel my body run and enjoy running to the music.*

Expecting but Not Caring About Sensations

Chapter 10 offers additional specific strategies for concerns about or an overfocus on the symptoms of exertion, but at this point we have a simple message: Feel the sensations of exercising, but don't get stuck paying attention *only* to these sensations. When you run, your heart will pound, you will sweat, your face may flush, your body may get hot, and you may have a wide variety of aches and pains in addition to feelings of fatigue. Expect to feel these sensations. When you get good at exercising, these sensations won't go away, but you will just no longer care about them. Given that this *not caring about* (or even looking forward to) these sensations is the endpoint of a good exercise habit, you might as well begin practicing this ability now.

When you exercise, be open to a wide range of experiences. Notice your feelings of breathlessness, notice the color of the tree off to your right, notice the sounds around you, notice the feel of your running stride, notice what you are daydreaming about, and keep running.

The limit to this approach is actually paying attention to pains or signs of injury. If there is a pebble in your shoe or your shoelaces are pinching, stop and correct the problem. If you feel you are having a knee problem or are experiencing odd muscle weakness or chest pain, consult a physician. The aim is to get good at tolerating everyday signs of exertion while also taking care of your body. Be sure to get answers to any questions you may have about odd or painful sensations or experiences during exercising.

Thoughts Immediately After Exercising

As we describe below, what you say to yourself after exercising will make a big difference in maintaining your exercise habit.

Rehearsal of Benefit

Exercising for a half-an-hour may have been hard, but it is important to ask yourself what was useful about it and to notice how you feel immediately afterwards (underscoring for yourself any immediate mood benefits). This sort of rehearsal of benefit is important for almost any situation requiring effort. Think of a work or school project where you had to apply yourself, push yourself, or otherwise put effort into finishing it. Recall the sense of relief and joy you may have felt at the completion. This joy, and making sure you feel it and remember it, is a primary factor in determining whether you feel motivated and competent the next time you need to do something hard.

Enjoying Your Success

Because exercising can be hard some days, and is at least taxing most days, you will need to make sure that you enjoy your successful exercise sessions each time they occur. Right after exercise, as you cool down, change clothes, or shower, we want you to mark your success by saying something like the following:

- *Wow, I did it!*
- *That was hard, and now I feel tired but good.*
- *I am tired, but I did something really useful for my mood.*
- *I attended to my body today, and my body carried me through the exercise.*
- *Good for me! I walked some, I ran some, but I exercised for a full half-hour.*
- *That was really hard; I really gave myself quite a workout. I can look forward to feeling the benefits of this later.*

I was unable to keep running. But the good news is, whether I ran or walked, I completed my 30 minutes of exercise.

I remember how I felt before the exercise session. I feel much better now. Not only do I feel more relaxed, I also feel very good about my accomplishment.

Thoughts Hours After Exercise

One strategy to help increase your motivation for exercising the next day is called echoing. "Echoing" is the process of making sure that a pleasant event has a recurring presence during the day. Particularly during periods where you might otherwise be daydreaming about problems, take a moment to reflect on (echo) your exercise success. Thoughts may include the following:

- *I did it! I got in exercise today to help my mood and body.*
- *I can still feel fatigue; I gave myself a good run today.*
- *This feeling in my legs means I am taking care of myself and using my body to help my mood.*
- *I was bothered by the feelings I had during exercise, but I really did it. I am getting stronger.*
- *I have gotten in three exercise sessions so far this week; I am really doing it—I am investing in my own future for a better mood and good health.*
- *Now that I've done several exercise sessions, I can tell that I love the feeling afterwards.*
- *It is great to see that such a small investment of time can have such a nice payoff.*

By paying attention to your periods of success, tracking them, and putting effort into repeating them, you will be helping create motivation for a lifelong health habit. Also, consider echoing all of the useful things you do every day as a way of life.

Hating Some Exercise Sessions

We want you to know for sure that you will HATE some of your exercise sessions. For example, some runs, for no reason that you can identify, will be lousy. On each step, your legs will feel like they are made of lead. You will feel like you have no energy. You will be paying attention to every breath. And all of the earlier advice on redirecting your attention to more pleasant things will fail. You will hate the run. This happens! But you will still get the benefits of exercise. And your next run may be terrific.

It is important to know that there is nothing about a few miserable exercise sessions that can defeat your ultimate success at becoming a regular exerciser. Expect some bad days, but still finish the exercise each session. You may walk instead of run, take extra breaks, scowl, and swear, but you can bounce back from these episodes. Tell yourself, "It happens. That was no fun, but I still treated my body well and will still get the benefits of whatever exercise I did." Then, expect that tomorrow's exercise session will be better.

Careful of the "Shoulds"

In the first chapter of this workbook, we recommended that you come to your new exercise program with fresh expectations. We did this to try to help you feel free from your own history of exercise successes or failures. One reason we did this is to help you be free of the "shoulds" surrounding exercise. "Shoulds" are statements about the way the world (or our workouts) should be based on some internal or external standard. Internal standards come from our own history, where we may decide that a run should be as fast as it was 5 or 10 years ago, or a 50-meter swim should have that smooth feeling of cutting through the water just like it did in college, or that a jump shot in basketball should go in the basket most of the time. External standards come from the demon of comparison—that you should lift as much, walk as fast, or serve as well as the person across the gym from you. Each of these "shoulds" detract from your ability to be in the moment and enjoy exercise, and they sap whatever achievement or joy you might be feeling by denigrating your performance relative to a standard from some other time or some other person. And we can admit that sometimes it is way too hard to step away from old standards based on who we used to be in a sport. For this reason, sometimes it is easier to begin your current routine with a program of exercise that is *not* what you used to do as a primary sport when younger. Starting new helps you get around old standards for your exercise performance, just in case those old standards feel too hard to challenge.

We would also like you to consider carefully how much you want to include competition in your exercise. Competition in a tennis or pickleball game can be terrific. Competition against your leaderboard score on the Peloton® can be motivating. But competition that turns into a perfectionistic "should" (a rigid demand rather than a fun challenge to try to win or beat an exercise standard) is usually destructive. When you are engaging in an exercise program, particularly for mental health benefits, you don't have to win and you don't have to beat your old time. What you have to do is make the exercise program enjoyable and sustainable so that you can get the benefits you want.

GOALS

- To determine if you are medically ready for an exercise program
- To find the right exercise activity for you
- To work toward the recommended dose of exercise
- To learn how to pace your exercise session
- To decide when to exercise
- To address possible barriers to exercise
- To use an exercise log to track your progress

OVERVIEW

This chapter gets you started thinking about which exercise activities might be right for you, including considering the desired duration and intensity of your exercise as well as how you can best schedule exercise sessions into your busy lifestyle.

Determining Readiness for an Exercise Program

Before starting your exercise program, we recommend that you work with your therapist to determine whether you need medical clearance. As an initial step, you should complete Worksheet 5.1: Physical Activity Readiness Questionnaire (PAR-Q), which provides screening items for health conditions that caution against starting exercise without physician approval. Worksheets can be found at the end of this chapter or can be accessed by searching for this book's title on the Oxford Academic platform, at academic.oup.com. In recent years, an expanded form of this questionnaire, the Physical Activity Readiness Questionnaire for Everyone (PAR-Q+), has been developed and can be found using an online search. Be sure to discuss the results of your PAR-Q or PAR-Q+ assessment and possible follow-up steps with your therapist.

Finding the Right Activity for You

One of the first choices in planning exercise is deciding what might be the most reasonable activity for you. As we have noted, walking and running are popular choices because they are readily available. Nonetheless, you and your therapist should consider other available alternatives. Worksheet 5.2: Selecting Activities lists some examples of moderate-intensity and vigorous-intensity activities. If you are interested in a more extensive list of activities with corresponding intensity, one is provided online by the Centers for Disease Control and Prevention at https://www.cdc.gov/nccdphp/dnpa/physical/pdf/pa_intensity_table_2_1.pdf. Note that the intensity of each activity listed in this document is expressed in METs (metabolic equivalency tasks). Activities associated with greater than 6 METs are vigorous in intensity; activities of 3 to 6 METs are moderate in intensity.

Working Toward the Public Health–Recommended Dose

Research to date is clear in showing mood benefits for exercise, and it appears that these benefits are better when you get a full dose of exercise. The best information on a full dose is provided by the Department of Health and Human Services. According to these guidelines, a full dose of health-giving aerobic exercise is:

1. Moderate-intensity aerobic exercise for at least 150 minutes (2 hours and 30 minutes) each week OR
2. Vigorous-intensity aerobic exercise for at least 75 minutes (1 hour and 15 minutes) each week.

Moderate-intensity aerobic exercise involves activities that *noticeably* increase your heart rate (e.g., brisk walking), whereas vigorous-intensity activity *substantially* increases your heart rate and causes you to breathe much faster (e.g., jogging). For reducing depression or anxiety, the literature supports programs of aerobic exercise done in bouts of at least 25 minutes on three to five days a week.

Determining Your Target Heart Rate

Perhaps the easiest method to determine the intensity of exercise is to simply measure your heart rate during the activity. The target heart rate that corresponds with moderate-intensity exercise is between 64% and 76% of the age-adjusted maximal heart rate (HR_{max}; 220 – age). Exercise intensity becomes vigorous when your heart rate ranges between 77% and 93% of your HR_{max}. Use the formulas provided in Exercise 5.1 to determine your target heart rate.

Initial Exercise Schedule

Naturally, you want to choose a starting point that will allow you to stay with your exercise habit. Our belief is that, to establish a strong exercise habit, there is no starting level that is too low. Walking several times a week, just to get in the habit of regular exercise, is a more reasonable alternative than overworking during an initial exercise attempt and being sore and resentful during the rest of the week. Start small and make your habit strong. Figure 5.1 presents a possible schedule for the initial weeks of your exercise program. As you can see, by gradually changing the intensity, duration, and frequency of your exercise sessions, you may take 3 or 4 weeks (or whatever you and your therapist decide) to get your activity schedule up to the recommended dose. Using Worksheet 5.3: Determining Your Initial Exercise Training Progression, you and your therapist should create a schedule to get you to your correct exercise dose. Remember that worksheets can be found at the end of this chapter or can

---

Exercise 5.1: Determining Target Heart Rate

Moderate-intensity exercise

Vigorous-intensity exercise

64% to 76% × (220 – your age) =_______% to _______%   77% to 93% × (220 – your age) =_______% to _______%

Week	Exercise intensity	Exercise duration	Exercise frequency
1	65% of HR_{max}	15 min	2 times per week
2	65–70% of HR_{max}	15–20 min	2–3 times per week
3	70–75% of HR_{max}	20–25 min	3–4 times per week
4	75–80% of HR_{max}	25–30 min	3–5 times per week

Figure 5.1

Sample Initial Exercise Training Progression

be accessed by searching for this book's title on the Oxford Academic platform, at academic.oup.com.

Pacing Your Exercise Session

In order to maximize your success with exercise and reduce the risk of injury, you should start your exercise session with a warm-up and finish it with a cool-down period. The warm-up period should last between 10 and 15 minutes and should begin with some low-intensity exercise (e.g., slow walking) followed by stretching activities. You should then slowly increase the intensity of your activity until it reaches the lower end of the target heart rate range for that session. Although it is often tempting to stop as soon as you have completed your scheduled activity, we recommend that you allow your body to gradually recover from the intense activity, so finish your routine by walking slowly for approximately 5 minutes followed by another 5 minutes of stretching.

When to Exercise

Chapter 3 provided you with information on the challenges and benefits that are associated with exercise at certain times of the day. Be sure to consider some of these challenges in relation to your personal schedule in deciding when to exercise. To start figuring this out, it is useful to have a clear notion of what your week is like and the natural periods when you are more or less busy or stressed. You may want to choose the higher-stress periods for exercise breaks, but we also understand that it is harder to fit in the time for exercise on those days. Use Worksheet 5.4: Daily Schedule Planner to write out your schedule of regularly occurring events at the present time, and then work with your therapist to pick times when exercise might best fit into your schedule.

Addressing Barriers to Exercise

As discussed in Chapters 3 and 4, motivating yourself to exercise may be particularly difficult at the beginning of an exercise-training program, when you haven't experienced any of the benefits. You may find that you don't have the time or it is inconvenient to exercise. You may also find exercise boring or have little confidence in your ability to be active, or you may even have concerns about getting injured. These barriers to exercise are common. Being aware of your perceived barriers and developing strategies to overcome them may help you be successful in making exercise part of your daily life.

Try to take a proactive approach in planning your weekly exercise program. As a first step, write down your exercise schedule for the week and list possible or anticipated barriers to completing this schedule (see Worksheet 5.5: Exercise Planning, located at the end of this chapter and also available by searching for this book's title on the Oxford Academic platform, at academic.oup.com). Then, create a list of possible strategies that you can use to overcome each barrier. It may be useful to enlist the help of your therapist or a friend in this process. They can help you be fair in assessing what stands in the way for you to become more active and can possibly offer some creative solutions to these barriers. Figure 5.2 shows a completed example of the Exercise Planning Worksheet.

Time Demands

We are used to the question, "When am I supposed to find time to exercise?" To address this question, you may need to keep a log of your time and activities to see just where your time is going. Pay particular attention to sedentary time. Data from the United States and from England suggest that screen time continues to account for a huge number of sedentary

Monday	Tuesday	Wednesday	Thursday
Activity: _Run_	Activity: _______	Activity: _Run_	Activity: _______
Intensity: _65% HR$_{max}$_	Intensity: _______	Intensity: _70% HR$_{max}$_	Intensity: _______
Duration: _25 min_	Duration: _______	Duration: _30 min_	Duration: _______
Friday	**Saturday**	**Sunday**	**SUMMARY**
Activity: _______	Activity: _Run_	Activity: _______	Intensity: _65–75%_
Intensity: _______	Intensity: _75% HR$_{max}$_	Intensity: _______	Duration: _25–40 min_
Duration: _______	Duration: _40 min_	Duration: _______	Frequency: _3_

Anticipated barriers	*Possible solutions*
1. Travel for work	1. Stay at a hotel that has exercise facilities
	2. Join a gym that has multiple locations in multiple cities
	3. Join the YMCA or YWCA
2. Lack of energy	1. Plan to exercise in the morning when I feel most energetic
	2. Remind myself that my energy increases with exercise
	3.

Figure 5.2

Example of a Completed Worksheet 5.5: Exercise Planning

hours each week in the lives of adults. If this is true for you, screen time would be an ideal time to target for change into exercise time.

Efficiency in exercise scheduling is also important. For example, make sure that a trip to the gym is scheduled when you are likely to be out driving already or is part of the commute to or from work. Also consider the role of brief workouts in your exercise routine. Although 40-minute workouts are a standard recommendation, it is also clear that even brief workouts (as little as 10 minutes) can provide benefit if summed into a fuller weekly dose of exercise (see below). You may also find that if you commit to just 10 minutes of exercise on your busiest days, you may enjoy the exercise break so much that you add an additional 10 or 20 minutes. Also, exercising for 10 minutes on your busiest days keeps you in the groove (thinking about the benefits of exercise and feeling like an "exerciser") for a longer workout the next day.

As first discussed in Chapter 3, this Exercise+ approach is also useful for managing some time challenges. If television time continues to be a barrier, consider watching TV during exercise using a stationary bike or treadmill supporting this Exercise+ strategy. If the need for family time is a barrier, consider family exercise: Can a climbing gym membership, a trip to the trampoline park, or evening walks satisfy some of the family time demands?

And don't forget the importance of habit. Once you begin to schedule in regular exercise, the rest of your schedule will adapt to your exercise times. Further, if you schedule your exercise as part of a regular weekly routine (same time, same place, etc.) you will find that it becomes easier and easier to get to your exercise and get it done. But don't take habit too far: Keep in mind that one key to enjoying exercise over the long term is knowing that your exercise routine does not have to remain the same. If there is a different time of day, or a different activity, or different clothes that can freshen up your enjoyment during exercise, make the change. Part of the process of starting a new exercise routine is finding a balance between (1) giving yourself enough time to get more comfortable with a new routine to make it yours, and (2) knowing that you may not find the right exercise activity on your first try and need an alternative program.

Use of Exercise Logs

The use of exercise logs (such as Worksheet 5.6: Exercise for Mood Log) can be helpful to keep your efforts, strategies, and achievements clear to you. In the beginning of your exercise program, these logs will be fairly detailed and have space for you to record not only your exercise but also the impact of exercise on your mood. Completing these logs after each exercise session should help you track your progress and see the mood benefits of your program. Use a new copy of the worksheet for each week of the first 6 weeks of your exercise program (or however long it takes you to get up to the public health–recommended dose). One copy of this worksheet appears at the end of this chapter, and additional copies can be accessed by searching for this book's title on the Oxford Academic platform, at academic.oup.com. An example of a completed worksheet is provided in Figure 5.3, showing results for a person relatively new (week 3) to an exercise-for-mood program.

	Day 1 Date:__/__	Day 2 Date:__/__	Day 3 Date:__/__	Day 4 Date:__/__	Day 5 Date:__/__	Day 6 Date:__/__	Day 7 Date:__/__
Day of the week	Monday	Tuesday	Wednesday	Thursday	Friday	Saturday	Sunday
Exercise completed (✓)	✓		✓			✓	✓
Time of day of exercise	7PM		7PM			11AM	1PM
Type of exercise completed	Aerobic Treadmill		Aerobic Treadmill			Aerobic Walking	Strength Weights
Intensity (%HR_{max})	119		123			136	
Duration (minutes)	20		25			29	47
Pre-exercise Feelings/Mood	3		2			6	5
Post-exercise Feelings/Mood	4		4			7	6

Figure 5.3

Example of Completed Worksheet 5.6: Exercise for Mood Log

If you are between the ages of 15 and 69, the PAR-Q will tell you if you should check with your doctor before engaging in physical activity. Common sense is your best guide when you answer these questions. Please read them carefully and answer each one honestly by checking Yes or No.

Yes No

☐ ☐ 1. Has your doctor ever said that you have a heart condition and that you should only do physical activity recommended by a doctor?

☐ ☐ 2. Do you feel pain in your chest when you do physical activity?

☐ ☐ 3. In the past month, have you had chest pain when you were not doing physical activity?

☐ ☐ 4. Do you lose your balance because of dizziness or do you ever lose consciousness?

☐ ☐ 5. Do you have a bone or joint problem (e.g., back, knee, or hip) that could be made worse by a change in your physical activity?

☐ ☐ 6. Is your doctor currently prescribing drugs for high blood pressure or heart condition?

☐ ☐ 7. Do you know of any other reason why you should not engage in physical activity?

*If you answered Yes to one or more questions, talk to your doctor **before** beginning a physical activity program.*

If you answered No to all questions, you can be reasonably sure that you can start becoming more physically active.

Source: Warburton, D. E., Jamnik, V. K., Bredin, S. S., McKenzie, D. C., Stone, J., Shephard, R. J., & Gledhill, N. (2011) Evidence-based risk assessment and recommendations for physical activity clearance: An introduction. *Applied Physiology, Nutrition, and Metabolism, 36*(Suppl 1), S1–S2. doi:10.1139/h11-060.

Check off or write in the activities that seem most fitting for your exercise interests.

Moderate-intensity exercise	**Vigorous-intensity exercise**
☐ Walking at 3–4 mph	☐ Jogging or running at >4.5 mph
☐ Bicycling on flat ground at 10–12 mph	☐ Bicycling on flat ground at >12 mph
☐ Swimming leisurely	☐ Swimming—moderate/hard
☐ Doubles tennis	☐ Cross-country skiing >2.5 mph
☐ Shooting baskets	☐ Rollerblading
☐ _______________________	☐ _______________________
☐ _______________________	☐ _______________________
☐ _______________________	☐ _______________________

Week	Exercise intensity	Exercise duration	Exercise frequency

	Morning	Mid-Day	Afternoon	Evening
Monday				
Tuesday				
Wednesday				
Thursday				
Friday				
Saturday				
Sunday				

Worksheet 5.5: Exercise Planning

Your exercise schedule for this week is:

Monday	Tuesday	Wednesday	Thursday
Activity: _____________	Activity: _____________	Activity: _____________	Activity: _____________
Intensity: ___________	Intensity: ___________	Intensity: ___________	Intensity: ___________
Duration: ___________	Duration: ___________	Duration: ___________	Duration: ___________
Friday	**Saturday**	**Sunday**	**SUMMARY**
Activity: _____________	Activity: _____________	Activity: _____________	**Intensity:** ___________
Intensity: ___________	Intensity: ___________	Intensity: ___________	**Duration:** ___________
Duration: ___________	Duration: ___________	Duration: ___________	**Frequency:** ___________

Anticipated barriers	*Possible solutions*
1.	1. 2. 3.
2.	1. 2. 3.

This log is to help you keep track of your exercise goals for mood by focusing on the importance of exercise several days a week.

Week Number__________

	Day 1 Date:__/__	Day 2 Date:__/__	Day 3 Date:__/__	Day 4 Date:__/__	Day 5 Date:__/__	Day 6 Date:__/__	Day 7 Date:__/__
Day of the week							
Exercise completed (✓)							
Time of day of exercise							
Type of exercise completed							
Intensity ($\%HR_{max}$)							
Duration (minutes)							
Pre-exercise feelings/mood							
Post-exercise feelings/mood							

GOALS

- To fine-tune your exercise program
- To enjoy your exercise treatment gains
- To learn how to bounce back from missed exercise sessions

OVERVIEW

The key to a successful exercise program over time is to plan for variation. Exercise that was right for you last month may not be right for you this month. This chapter contains information on how to adapt your exercise program to fit your current interests and needs.

Fine-Tuning Your Exercise Program

Once you have worked up to the minimum public health–recommended dose of exercise, your task becomes finding ways to continue to exercise. The aim is for exercise to become a stronger habit and a regular part of your ongoing routine. Following the first weeks of training, it will be useful to consider things you can do to make exercise an easier and better part of your routine. Do there need to be any changes in the timing of your exercise? Now that you are not so new to the program, are there other people you may want to involve in your exercise habit? At this point, we

suggest that you review Chapters 1, 3, and 4 to see if there are additional
supports you would like to put in place for your exercise routine.

Focusing on Your Individual Needs

Now is also an excellent time to make sure you are fine-tuning your exercise program to your individual needs:

- Chapter 8 provides additional information on the use of exercise as part of treatment for depression.
- Chapter 9 extends this information to apply to bipolar disorder and provides additional ideas for working with your clinical team.
- Chapter 10 is important to review if you are exercising as part of a program to manage anxiety or panic.
- Chapter 11 focuses on exercise for cognitive enhancement, such as improving your memory.
- Chapter 12 integrates Chapters 8 through 11 with a focus on psychological resilience.
- Chapter 13 covers exercise for smoking cessation.

These chapters offer ideas on how to change or add to your personal exercise routine to get additional cognitive or mood benefits.

Varying Intensity, Duration, and Frequency of Exercise

Continue to plan how you may want to change your exercise prescription
by varying one or more of the following three exercise parameters:

1. Intensity (the target heart rate)
2. Duration (minutes per session)
3. Frequency (number of sessions per week)

You or your therapist may want to make changes in these parameters to
help you better achieve your mood and fitness goals. If so, using Worksheet
6.1: Your Updated Exercise Prescription, write down your revised exercise
goals in the space provided. Worksheets can be found at the end of this
chapter or can be accessed by searching for this book's title on the Oxford
Academic platform, at academic.oup.com.

For management of mood and anxiety disorders in general, the public health–recommended dose of exercise should meet your needs. The exception to this general rule is that for the treatment of panic disorder, you want to make sure you exercise at a sufficient intensity to create the bodily symptoms of exertion. (Look at Figure 10.4 on p. 84 of this workbook for an example of how to do this.) Completing at least a 25-minute bout of exercise of this intensity three times a week will help you achieve a healthy dose of exercise while also making sure you become comfortable with stronger sensations of exertion—a goal we discuss in detail in Chapter 10. Use your time with your therapist to discuss your thoughts about and experiences with exercise and the changes you note relative to mood or anxiety symptoms.

Expanding your workout parameters can also add more fun to your exercise routines. As you establish a physical activity habit, you will likely make changes to the specific weekly program. You may want to add new exercises or plan for hard versus easy exercise sessions to create diversity in your routine. Making sure that you have diversity in your exercise experiences will help keep your exercise program interesting.

Keep in mind that pleasure during exercise is a strong predictor of whether you stay with exercise over the longer term. Because we do want you to keep working out over the longer term, let us ask: What can be done to increase your sense of pleasure during exercise? In answering this question, please think about not only your core exercise activity—whether you walk, play tennis, swim, etc.—but also what can be combined with the activity to increase pleasure. For example:

- Does your music need to be different, or is it time to try audiobooks?
- Do you need new workout partners, or can you involve your friends or family in the workout?
- Is your pleasure being lessened by what you are paying attention to during the exercise?
- Are you thinking about your sore left knee or all the things you need to do later in the day?
- Can you instead pay attention to how lovely the trees look this time of year?

It is important that you keep your attention on the benefits you are attaining with exercise. During and after any given exercise session, make sure you reflect on the gains you are receiving. For example:

- What are the ways in which you feel better?
- Are you noticing changes in the way you react to stress?
- Have others in your life commented on differences in your mood or in the quality of interactions with you?
- Do you find you have more energy or sleep better due to exercise?
- Has your attention or memory improved?
- Has your sense of the seasons or your town or city changed because exercise gets you outside?
- Have you developed new friendships because of exercise?

Noticing and enjoying these changes will help you settle into your exercise routine and acknowledge your achievements. Don't forget to congratulate yourself for whatever fitness level you have achieved so far in this program.

Managing Low-Motivation Moments

Sometimes the notion of a full workout seems too daunting to face. Let's be clear: You do not always need to push yourself to do a complete workout. Make sure you save up some very brief workouts for your low- or no-motivation days. Just 10 minutes of working out might be all you can do for a given day (and 10 minutes of sit-ups, push-ups, or a bike ride really is a workout that adds nicely to your weekly totals). Indeed, commercial apps from a variety of companies (e.g., Peloton®) offer 5- and 10-minute strength workouts as well as 10-minute aerobic workouts, helping legitimize this approach to adding up your total dose of exercise over time. Also, never underestimate how a brief workout can transform how you feel in the moment and how it may help you feel like doing a full workout tomorrow (because the 10-minute workout kept you feeling athletic and caring about your body and mood). Finally, it bears repeating that it is not uncommon for people to commit to just 10 minutes, but then feel like completing a longer workout once they are in the swing of things.

It is natural to miss sessions of exercise from time to time. Perhaps the most important aspect of establishing a longer-term exercise habit is becoming good at getting yourself right back into an exercise routine after a missed session. You will need to be especially wary of the bad coaching (what you might think to yourself) that can happen after a missed session. This bad coaching (doom-saying) takes a simple miss and translates it into a prescription for exercise failure. Such bad coaching includes the following thoughts:

- *I missed my exercise; I knew I could not stay with it.*
- *Regular exercise is just too hard; why bother?*
- *I wrecked my benefits already; there is no point in continuing.*
- *I missed exercise all this week; I might as well just give up.*

Alternative and useful coaching for missed sessions includes the following:

- *It is a challenge to keep a perfect exercise schedule; no reason to beat myself up. I just need to get back on track with even a short exercise session.*
- *Making sure I exercise tomorrow will make it easier to get back to my full routine next week.*
- *I am doing this for my mood; feeling low or unmotivated is exactly the reason to exercise.*
- *I like feeling in shape, and if I exercise later today, I get to keep and extend this feeling.*
- *I have to remember to exercise first, and expect to feel like exercising only after I am back on track.*

Also, to help yourself return from a lapse, you may want to look through some of your original motivations for exercise (from Chapter 1) as well as review some of your entries in Worksheet 5.6: Exercise for Mood Log. Seeing some of your recorded mood benefits is a nice way to enhance your motivation to get right back to a scheduled workout. Finally, you might want to contact a member of your support team; perhaps a workout with a friend or family member would help the next exercise session feel even better.

Worksheet 6.1: Your Updated Exercise Prescription

Use this worksheet to consider how you might want to modify your exercise program given your current progress and interests.

Week	Exercise intensity	Exercise duration	Exercise frequency

<table>
<tr><td>CHAPTER 7</td><td>Extending Your Exercise Program—Enjoyable Activities and Sleep</td></tr>
</table>

GOALS

- To keep a regular activity schedule
- To add more pleasant activities into your schedule
- To improve sleep quality

OVERVIEW

To help you get the most out of this program, this chapter discusses how to enhance your enjoyable activities and how to improve your sleep to strengthen your well-being from exercise.

Keeping a Regular Activity Schedule

Your exercise program is designed to provide you with a natural and effective mood lift. To make the most of this mood lift, it is important to provide yourself with a balance of activities that are pleasurable and that lead to a sense of accomplishment. In particular, you may notice that your fitness gains from regular exercise are opening new doors for you in terms of pleasurable activities. For example, once in better shape, it may be tempting to say "yes" to that invitation to ride bikes along the beach or go for a brief hike with friends or try out that yoga class. That is, as you progress with regular exercise, you have new possibilities for recreation opening up for you. As part of this process, continue to think about how you also want to "trade up" to more social or more fun exercise and life-engagement options as you meet your initial exercise goals for mood, anxiety, or cognition. Your progression may look something like this:

> Initiate exercise with slow walking ⇨ become comfortable with walking briskly ⇨ start a run/walk program ⇨ say "yes" to an invitation to try pickleball ⇨ start a regular doubles tennis program.

At every point in this transition, remember to continue a program of warming up and cooling down so that your body can adapt well to new exercise options. And please complement new exercise options with a broader menu of non-exercise pleasant events. As you did with exercise, you can also use Worksheet 5.4: Daily Schedule Planner (located near the end of Chapter 5) to help you structure a personalized weekly activity pattern that works for you. The first step in adding pleasant events into your life is to think about some of the enjoyable activities that you used to do or that you want to do. Once you identify these activities, write them on Worksheet 7.1: Valued Activities. Worksheets can be found at the end of this chapter or can be accessed by searching for this book's title on the Oxford Academic platform, at academic.oup.com.

Increasing Pleasant Activities

As exercise and activity increase as part of your exercise program, your desire for pleasant events may increase as well. Use Worksheet 5.4: Daily Schedule Planner (from Chapter 5) to better understand your average weekly schedule and to consider what changes you might like to make. Strive for a balance of regularly scheduled small activities or events to help you feel good. These events can be simple pleasant events (lunch with a friend, time for a hobby, a regular dinner out or movie night, etc.) as well as those activities that give you a sense of achievement (gardening, cleaning off your desk, finishing a project, etc.). As you take time to think about and schedule regular involvement in pleasant activities, consider the list of potentially pleasurable activities shown on Worksheet 7.2: Pleasant Events List. The value of this list is in encouraging you to think about a range of pleasant activities. Engaging in rewarding activities on a regular basis serves as a buffer against stress. Note that many of these activities involve physical activity, and hence many of these may be easier or more pleasurable to complete as you become more fit.

As you start and work to maintain your program of exercise, it is helpful to also get the most out of your sleep time. Exercise will naturally help you feel nicely fatigued (physical fatigue feels different than mental fatigue) and ready to sleep. To enhance this process, it is important to make sure you don't have any bad sleep habits that may be reducing the quality of your sleep time. The following tips will—in general—maximize the quality of your sleep.

Good Sleep Strategies

- Eliminate stress in the bedroom. Discussions about your life or family issues or evening work (e.g., paying bills and reading documents for work) should not take place in bed or in the bedroom. Save the bedroom for bed activities. Worry or work at a desk, not in bed.
- Give yourself time to unwind before sleep. Make sure the last hour of activity before bedtime is relatively passive. Do not pay bills, do not work out life problems, and do not plan your workday just before going to bed; save these activities for earlier in the day when you are fresher. Before sleep, choose activities that are pleasant and take very little effort (e.g., watching television, reading, and talking). Go to bed only after you have had a chance to unwind and feel more like sleeping.
- Use a regular daytime cycle to help with nighttime sleep. Avoid taking naps during the day. Use regular exercise (at least 3 hours before bedtime) to help increase sleep and induce normal fatigue. One way to establish a regular time for falling asleep is to have a regular time for waking up. Setting your alarm clock to a reasonable time and maintaining it throughout the week (including the weekend) will eventually be helpful in stabilizing your sleep time.
- Reduce caffeine use (certainly limit caffeine use after noon), and be wary of drinking alcohol or smoking within several hours of bedtime.
- If you have sleep problems, be careful of trying too hard to get to sleep. Trying hard to get to sleep often has the opposite effect: It wakes a person up with feelings of frustration and anger. Instead, try to enjoy being in bed and resting, even if sleep does not come. Direct your attention to how comfortable you are in bed (how

the pillow feels or how good it feels to lie down and stretch), how
relaxed your muscles feel, and how you can let your thoughts drift.
If sleep does not come in a reasonable time, get out of bed and do
a calm activity in another room. Return to bed only when you feel
sleepy.

- Use muscle relaxation techniques in bed. Relaxation scripts can
be found with a quick internet search, and many are available on
YouTube or from app stores. Find a version you like and use it to
feel even more comfortable in bed. Remember, the goal is not to
"compete to go to sleep" but to become very comfortable in bed so
that sleep comes naturally.

Worksheet 7.1: Valued Activities

For each of the categories below, please think about the activities that would add meaning to your life. This list may also include things that you have wanted in your life in the past but did not have the time or opportunity to pursue. Please add these activities to the spaces provided.

Social Activities

____

____

____

Recreation/Entertainment

____

____

____

Relationship Activities

____

____

____

Hobbies

____

____

____

Volunteer Activities

____

____

____

Work-Related Activities

____

____

____

The following list is designed to stimulate ideas for activities that may increase your weekly pleasure level as well as provide stress-buffering effects. In considering the list, think of the <u>variations on themes</u> that may make an activity especially rewarding. For example, adding little things to a regular activity— buying your favorite childhood candy at the movie theater or fixing a cup of tea to drink while reading a novel—can help transform an experience by evoking past pleasant memories.

As you go through the list, check off those activities of most interest to you:

- ☐ Go fishing in a local stream or pond
- ☐ Call two friends and go bowling
- ☐ Play with a Frisbee
- ☐ Take a kid to mini golf
- ☐ Take a yoga class
- ☐ Go to an indoor rock-climbing center— take a lesson
- ☐ Build a snow fort and have a snowball fight
- ☐ Walk in the snow and listen to your footsteps
- ☐ Catch snowflakes in your mouth
- ☐ Sign up for a sculpting class
- ☐ Bake a cake
- ☐ Draw
- ☐ Paint (oils, acrylics, watercolor)
- ☐ Climb a tree
- ☐ Go for an evening drive
- ☐ Go to a drive-in movie
- ☐ See a movie
- ☐ Volunteer to work at a soup kitchen
- ☐ Join a Friday night event at a museum
- ☐ Write a letter to a friend
- ☐ Sing a song
- ☐ Read the newspaper in a coffee shop
- ☐ Schedule a kissing-only date with your romantic partner
- ☐ Order hot chocolate in a restaurant
- ☐ Buy flowers for the house
- ☐ Get a massage
- ☐ Reread a book you read in high school or college
- ☐ Bake cookies for a neighbor
- ☐ Have a garage sale (perhaps with a neighbor)
- ☐ Buy a spool of wire and make a sculpture
- ☐ Go to an art museum and find one piece you really like
- ☐ Buy a magazine on a topic you know nothing about
- ☐ Polish all of your shoes
- ☐ Buy a new plant
- ☐ Clean out a closet
- ☐ Write a letter to the editor of the local newspaper
- ☐ Repaint a table or a shelf
- ☐ Play a musical instrument
- ☐ Take an art class
- ☐ Walk a dog
- ☐ Volunteer to walk dogs for a local animal shelter
- ☐ Play with children
- ☐ Visit a pet shop and look at the animals
- ☐ Sit in the sun
- ☐ Sit on a porch swing
- ☐ Go for a hike
- ☐ Learn to knit
- ☐ Do a crossword puzzle (each day for a week)
- ☐ Go out for an ice cream sundae
- ☐ Rent a garden plot at a local farm or community space
- ☐ Grill dinner in the back yard
- ☐ Take a bubble bath at night with candles around the tub

- ☐ Have a picnic at a park with a friend
- ☐ Have a tea party on your or your neighbor's front porch
- ☐ Go bird/nature watching
- ☐ Read a book under a tree
- ☐ Organize photos/vinyl record collection
- ☐ Write poetry
- ☐ Join a choir or singing group
- ☐ Do Sudoku puzzles
- ☐ Put on some dance music and dance in your living room
- ☐ Sign up for a class at the local community college or center
- ☐ Go to a diner for breakfast
- ☐ Devote a meal to cooking red, white, and blue foods
- ☐ Plan an affordable three-day vacation
- ☐ Start a collection of heart-shaped rocks
- ☐ Find your top three favorite videos on YouTube and share them with a friend
- ☐ Woodworking—build a table or a chair
- ☐ Create a playlist of your favorite movie music
- ☐ Take a dance class
- ☐ Learn to fold dollar bills into origami creatures
- ☐ Soak your feet in warm water
- ☐ Learn to juggle
- ☐ Clean and polish the inside of your car
- ☐ Go to a concert
- ☐ Meditate
- ☐ Organize a weekly game of cribbage or bridge
- ☐ Look at a map
- ☐ Plan a drive in the country
- ☐ Sew some napkins
- ☐ Make a pizza and bake it
- ☐ Buy a cookbook and make three new meals
- ☐ Read a novel
- ☐ Listen to your favorite song from high school . . . really loudly
- ☐ Make a scrapbook
- ☐ Read travel books about places you've always wanted to visit (and maybe plan a visit!)
- ☐ Play charades
- ☐ Go to the beach
- ☐ Go to the zoo
- ☐ Start writing a journal
- ☐ Play pub trivia
- ☐ Learn a new language
- ☐ Take a photo every day for a week
- ☐ Have a poker night
- ☐ Play horseshoes
- ☐ Go to a sporting event
- ☐ Play ping-pong
- ☐ Invite friends over for board games
- ☐ Invite friends over, make popcorn, and stream a movie
- ☐ Attend a local art event (a dance performance, a play, an art show opening)
- ☐ Go to a comedy club
- ☐ Join a book club
- ☐ Join an after-school program to mentor children
- ☐ Lie by a pool/river/lake/beach
- ☐ Take a historic tour of your city
- ☐ Get dressed up and go out for dinner with your romantic partner or friends
- ☐ Have a neighborhood barbeque
- ☐ Play video games

GOALS

- To learn about the thinking patterns that accompany depression
- To take advantage of the beneficial effects of exercise
- To use self-coaching
- To use your support team
- To sustain and increase your activity level

OVERVIEW

This chapter is designed to support you in using your exercise program to target depression. In addition to providing information about the nature of depression, this chapter includes specific exercises to complement your exercise program for mood.

Model of Depression

Depression is much more than the sad or blue mood people sometimes experience when they have had a bad day. Major depression is a medical disorder that is characterized by a slew of symptoms that are present daily or nearly every day for at least 2 weeks. Symptoms of depression include those listed in Worksheet 1.1: Symptoms to Be Targeted by Exercise in Chapter 1: blue mood, lack of interest, feelings of guilt, low energy, disrupted appetite, agitation or difficulties moving, sleep disruptions, and, at times, suicidal thoughts. Some or all of these symptoms may be present during depression, and their severity can make it difficult to function in life.

Negative Thinking

Depression, like many psychiatric disorders, involves a number of self-perpetuating cycles. The low mood leads to more negative thinking patterns and expectations of failure and disappointment. For example, when depressed, it is common for people to have negative thoughts about the following:

- Oneself (*I blew it*; *I am no good*; *It never works out for me*; *Look at me, I am such a loser!*)
- Others (*He does not care about me*; *They don't like me*)
- The future (*It won't work out*; *There is no point*)
- Ongoing goals, including one's exercise program (*Exercise is doing nothing for me*; *There is no point in continuing*)

This type of thinking can worsen a depressed mood, increase feelings of hopelessness, and decrease engagement in useful behaviors and problem-solving. Not only will you have thoughts of this kind, but these thoughts will also *feel* more true during periods of stress and depression. Moreover, it is important to remember that *negative thoughts do not have to be true to have a powerful effect on your emotions*. It is important that you treat your thoughts as rough guesses about the world rather than as true statements of what is going on. And these guesses have as much to do with your current mood state and thinking habits as they do about external reality.

Repetitive Thoughts

Another feature of thinking patterns in depression is the focus on repetitive thoughts. If you have depression, you may find that you turn the same thought over and over again (ruminations) with no useful outcome. When cognitively ruminating, you never get a break from your problems, and have little ability to notice that better, less painful things may be going on in your life. Thinking this way can be like putting your tongue in the socket of a missing tooth: it hurts, but at the same time, it feels almost irresistible to check and see if it still hurts! Because of this, ruminations can be a strong force in keeping your mood low.

One useful aspect of hard aerobic exercise is that it is very difficult to keep ruminating during and after the exercise. In fact, one of the early effects you may notice that exercise such as running has on depression is that, during the last half of your exercise period, your mind becomes quiet. Instead of having ongoing repetitive negative thoughts, you may begin to notice other feelings and events—the sky, the trees, your music. With ongoing running, your mind may return to how you are when not depressed.

This program wants you to be prepared to take advantage of this effect. When exercising to help relieve depression, be prepared to have a rumination-free period during your exercise session. Prior to running, for example, you may want to instruct yourself, "This run is a time when I *do not* have to think about how I feel or focus on my negative thoughts. This will be an opportunity to just be in the moment, feeling whatever I feel during the run, and enjoying my music and the sights along my running route."

Coaching

Also, when exercising to relieve depression, it will be important for you to put in extra effort to coach yourself effectively. Because of depression, you may have a number of negative and motivation-sapping thoughts:

- *Why bother? Nothing is going to help this depression.*
- *Who cares! I feel so bad already; exercise will just make me feel worse.*
- *I just want to be in bed; I will run tomorrow.*

When you have these kinds of thoughts, the goal is to be effective at *listening to the chatter but exercising anyway.*

When you are depressed, your thoughts will naturally become overly negative, and you will have to be very careful about placing too much belief in them. Instead, you will need to be a good coach to yourself around the negative throughs that come in depression: *notice* your thoughts, *observe* how the thoughts make you feel, and gently *redirect* your thoughts when you find they are not useful for helping you live your life. Negative thoughts are so common in depression that you may want to practice treating some of your negative thoughts like they are wayward children.

You understand why the thoughts want to go wandering off in the direction in which they go, but you don't need to follow them (with your behavior). For example, when faced by negative thoughts about running, you may want to say the following to yourself:

Yes, it is possible that . . .

- *Exercise won't work for me.*
- *I should just stay in bed.*
- *Lying down or watching television now would be comforting.*

But now is my scheduled exercise time. I will see what I feel like doing after I exercise.

Using Your Support Team

When exercising to help treat your depression, you will want to use every available situational support. Ask one of your support team members (look back at Worksheet 1.3: Selecting Members of Your Support Team in Chapter 1) to encourage you to exercise. Be specific in telling this person how you want coaching: "Please give me a call weekly and ask me how my exercise program is going; I like the idea of having someone to talk to about it" or "I would love it if you could walk with me weekly. I am trying to keep up with a new exercise program. Knowing that we could walk together would really help me stay with it, and you will get the benefits as well."

Using an Exercise+ Approach

When exercising for mood, we would like you to see what sort of Exercise+ strategies work best for you. Organize your exercise equipment in one place—we don't want you to miss an exercise session because you can't find your left running shoe. And speaking of shoes, would it be useful to put a reminder of why you are exercising in your left shoe—a note stating "mood?" Also, is there an audiobook or a promise of good music that will make it easier for you to get to your exercise? If you can, pick a podcast, audiobook, or playlist of music that you save as special for your workout time. Then look forward to having a break to enjoy that program while you are doing your exercise.

Or figure out which exercise days you are going to schedule with a friend or family member. Having someone expecting you on the running route is a great way to make sure you reliably make your exercise time. You may want to refer back to previous chapters to be ready for some strong self-coaching to get yourself to your exercise (Chapter 4) at the dose that is most recommended for mental health benefits (Chapter 5). Then you can allow the natural variations in exercise—good days, bad days, strong workouts, and "cheat days"—that affect all of us working to integrate regular exercise into our lifestyle.

Sustaining and Increasing Activity Levels

One effect of depression is a reduced activity level. And with reduced activity, individuals with depression are cut off from the very activities that could help restore their mood. In addition to the direct lifts in mood that can come after a session of exercise, merely sustaining your activity levels (by exercising several times a week) can help extend exercise's antidepressant effects.

To achieve a balanced lifestyle, exercise should be one part of a series of mood-enhancing activities. Recommendations for this goal are provided in Chapter 7. After you have established a regular exercise habit, add in other pleasurable events that help promote a positive mood. Use Worksheet 7.2: Pleasant Events List (found in Chapter 7) as well as Worksheet 5.4: Daily Schedule Planner (found in Chapter 5) to schedule these buffering events. We call them "buffering events" because they can help buffer the effects of a low mood or a stressful week. Having something to look forward to, even if you feel blue, and participating in these activities can have powerful effects on reducing depression.

"Leaning in" to the Mood Effects of Exercise

Some of the mood benefits of exercise emerge within 20 minutes of a good aerobic workout. Look for these effects. That is, after you have a chance to cool down and recover (e.g., after you have stopped sweating and feel more comfortable), take a moment to check on your mood: Do you feel calmer and better? And notice that you can feel good while feeling tired from the workout. Lean in to these feelings, coaching yourself around how your exercise is useful for you. For example, you may think, "It was hard to start the exercise, but I really do feel better now" or "My mind feels clearer and I feel more at peace. I really helped myself by getting myself to exercise."

In addition to feeling some of these benefits after most exercise sessions (but not every single one), the mood benefits of exercise increase across your weeks of regular exercise. Most of the studies of the antidepressant effects of exercise examined results after 12 weeks (assuming you are exercising around four times a week), with evidence that the mood benefits of exercise increase week by week across this time period. We don't know what your particular pattern of improvement may be, and we certainly don't expect you to feel good after every exercise session, but in general it pays to expect increasing benefits over the time you stay in your exercise program.

- To learn about bipolar disorder and its treatment
- To use exercise as an additional treatment for bipolar disorder
- To challenge loaded words and phrases

This chapter extends exercising for mood to the management of bipolar disorder. Information is provided on bipolar disorder and the role of exercise and activity balance in helping to manage this disorder.

About Bipolar Disorder and Its Treatment

Bipolar disorder is a relatively common psychiatric disorder that in its classic form affects 1% to 2% of the population. Bipolar disorder is characterized by recurrent episodes of mood disturbance that occurs on two "poles": periods of depression and periods of mood elevation, where individuals feel so hyper that they feel they are not their normal selves. These periods of elevated mood meet criteria for mania when the moods are accompanied by symptoms such as racing thoughts, inflated self-esteem, decreased need for sleep, and over-participation in activities (gambling, risky sex, extramarital affairs, investments, etc.) that have a high potential for harm. There are a number of subtypes of bipolar disorder that are defined by the degree of elevated mood (full mania or a less severe version of mania called "hypomania"). Likewise, people with bipolar disorder may differ in whether the disorder is characterized by the down periods—the depressions that define the other pole of bipolar disorder. In most cases, at any given time it is more common to find individuals suffering from the depressive symptoms than the manic symptoms in bipolar disorder. However, because of the cycle of the disorder, treatment efforts in bipolar disorder are aimed at eliminating the current mood episode as well as preventing the next one.

Treatment for Bipolar Disorder

For decades, the dominant treatment for bipolar disorder was an exclusive focus on medications using a variety of mood-stabilizing, antipsychotic, antidepressant, and anti-anxiety medications to manage the disorder. Recently, however, a variety of studies have shown that certain types of psychotherapy can have powerful effects on treating bipolar disorder as well as helping prevent relapse. Certain types of psychotherapies for depression, such as cognitive-behavioral therapy, have been applied to bipolar depression with promising results. These findings give us some confidence that exercise interventions, shown to be effective for treating depression, will have similar effects on bipolar depression.

There are other reasons to expect that exercise may help with bipolar disorder:

1. There is evidence that programmed exercise can reduce stress and anxiety among individuals with bipolar disorder, and both stress and anxiety are related to a higher number and greater severity of mood episodes.
2. The stability of sleep–wake patterns is important in the management of bipolar disorder, and exercise offers benefits for sleep quality and stability.
3. Treatments for bipolar disorder frequently include programs to structure sleep, wake, and activity cycles, and exercise can play an important role in those treatments.
4. Many people with bipolar disorder experience periods of irritability and anger, and studies have shown less anger and cynical distrust

among individuals who exercise frequently. So for a person with bipolar disorder, exercise may help calm their feelings of irritability and anger.

5. Some of the medications used to help manage mood in bipolar disorder can lead to significant weight gain. In response to this challenge, a number of specialty clinics for bipolar disorder are beginning to consider lifestyle management programs that offer exercise to clients who need to take these medications. Hence, exercise, in addition to providing direct effects for mood management, can also provide benefit by reducing some of the side effects (weight gain) of other treatments for bipolar disorder.

Using Exercise in the Management of Bipolar Disorder

Medications are still the core treatment for bipolar disorder, and exercise is a supplement to—not a replacement for—this treatment. Exercise provides an additional and active element of treatment that clients can make their own and apply on a near-daily basis. For this reason, exercise is sometimes an especially pleasing option for people with bipolar disorder because it involves such active and personal effort as compared to medication use alone. Indeed, bipolar disorder is one of those conditions where medication, psychotherapy, and exercise together can be an extremely effective combination.

An additional element of an exercise program if you have bipolar disorder is the focus on *balance*. Exercise should become a regular part of a near-daily routine. It should be done regardless of your ups and down in mood, and you should view exercise as the time of the day to "lock in" moderation. The goal is for exercise to work like clockwork in your schedule, providing a break that you can rely upon.

Also, you can use your monitoring of your exercise as a way to keep track of your mood. Moderation is the key, and you will need to monitor urges to over-exercise or skip exercise. These urges may be part of a normal pattern of wanting a break from a routine, but with bipolar disorder it pays to also ask the question: "Is this part of my normal variability in interest, or is this a sign that I should watch whether this is a symptom of a mood episode?" In either case, early intervention (calling your therapist and discussing options) is especially important for the overall management of bipolar disorder. In addition to a program of exercise, we strongly recommend that you create a balanced and rewarding activity schedule, as discussed in Chapter 7.

Loaded Words and Phrases

The previous chapter gave recommendations to *notice* your thoughts, *observe* how the thoughts make you feel, and gently *redirect* your thoughts. For the management of bipolar disorder, you will also want to notice the form your thoughts take, with particular attention to the presence of "loaded words." These are words or phrases that evoke lots of emotion despite being inaccurate. They are exaggerations of everyday outcomes, and they have the effect of making us feel worse than we need to feel. With loaded words, minor social mishaps become "disasters," a less-than-optimal outcome becomes a "failure," and mistakes become evidence that we are "so stupid." The consequence of these thoughts is that everyday events feel more dire and depressing. Also, when you are feeling more down, you will tend to use thoughts like these when thinking about yourself.

This program wants to make you aware of these types of thoughts so that when you hear them, you can redirect yourself toward more accurate thinking. You can do this by challenging your assessment (*What do I really mean by "disaster"? What about this situation really deserves that label?*). The goal is to help you react realistically to situations rather than reacting to overly emotional descriptions of the situation. Use Exercise 9.1: Replacing Loaded Words and Phrases, as needed.

A Balanced Lifestyle

Exercising for bipolar disorder provides a weekly opportunity to practice balance. Because of its core focus on regular activity, exercise provides a balance to spending too much time in your head or getting stuck on the couch. Exercise also provides great training in having a balanced schedule, with workout days and rest days. Exercise can encourage a balanced "here and now" mental attitude as part of the practice of staying in the moment during exercise and seeing what you can notice to best entertain yourself. Finally, exercise is not just for helping with a mood episode; it is also a tool to stabilize your mood for the long term—completing exercise as a way of life regardless of whether you feel down, hyped, or in a period of recovery. For this reason, Chapter 12 on resilience is a natural complement to this chapter, providing an additional focus on preventing relapse and enhancing well-being.

Think back on a time you used some of the loaded words shown below and give yourself some practice writing out more accurate appraisals.

Appraisal with loaded words	Accurate appraisal and planning
It was _______________________	I don't think the event went well because of (be
■ A disaster	specific) _________________________________
■ A nightmare	____
■ Terrible	____
■ _________________________	
	Next time it would be better if I (be specific) _________
I was a ____________________	
■ Failure	____
■ Loser	____
■ Reject	____
■ _________________________	

GOALS

- To recognize and defer worries
- To learn about panic attacks and panic disorder
- To learn about the treatment for panic disorder
- To apply exercise to panic disorder

OVERVIEW

This chapter opens with information about some of the common patterns underlying anxiety and panic disorders. Exercise can be used to address these patterns, in part by capitalizing on the ways in which regular exercise helps you become comfortable with the rapid heart rate, rapid breathing, sweating, and host of other bodily sensations that go along with vigorous exercise. These sensations from exercise can be used to help you react differently to the nervous system (autonomic) arousal that is part of anxiety disorders and panic.

Introduction

We have all had those moments when we just can't get worried thoughts out of our head. They come in over and over again. Worry is a self-perpetuating process. Worrying about problems increases feelings of stress and anxiety, and these feelings make our worries and anxiety-provoking thoughts *feel* more true.

When symptoms of stress and anxiety are strong—when we feel a tight chest, sweaty palms, queasy stomach, racing heart, and dizziness—anxious thoughts can be particularly hard to dismiss. We can lose control of useful problem-solving. We lose perspective! Thoughts may take on a life of their own, and it is hard to turn away from anxious ruminations. Exercise may be the perfect action to take in these moments. Exercise can help you reset your mood and thoughts and provide you with several hours of calmer and clearer thinking after you exercise. The key is remembering to use exercise at these moments.

Recognizing and Deferring Worries

Anxiety-inducing thoughts are often in the form of "What if . . . " (*What if I get fired? What if they break up with me? What if the kids get sick? What if she is mad? What if the report is flawed? What if things get worse?*). In anxiety conditions typified by worry, it is common for individuals to bring up an anxiety-provoking thought, experience the emotional cost of the thought (increased anxiety and tension), and then shift to an alternative thought. The process looks something like what we see in Figure 10.1.

In many cases, individuals under stress just need a break so that they can regain perspective rather than being caught in a cycle of unproductive/anxious thinking. An exercise session can be just the thing to give you a break from these thoughts and—most importantly—give you perspective.

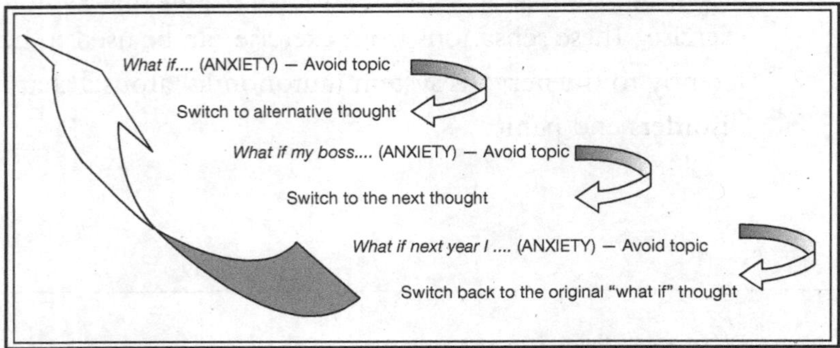

Figure 10.1
Diagram of the Worry Process

You can then engage in productive problem-solving (actually thinking about solutions rather than ruminating about potential problems).

However, when you are in the middle of stress or anxiety, you may not be at a point in the day when you can just take an exercise break. Instead, you will need to practice *deferring* worry and rumination until you can get perspective. When you feel yourself in a loop of anxious thoughts, we want you to ask yourself, "Do I really need to think about this now, and is my thinking leading to solutions?" You may want to coach yourself by saying something like the following:

I don't need to think about this all the time. It feels good to have a break from these thoughts. What can I notice in the here and now that is more pleasant than turning over "what if" thoughts in my mind?

Then, during your next exercise session, allow yourself to use your exercise and physical exertion to provide you with a period of perspective. Your goal is to use the natural effects of exercise to induce a worry-free period and to create a sense of calmness to help you stay worry-free for hours after exercise.

Panic Attacks and Panic Disorder

At times, anxiety comes on so suddenly and so strongly that it becomes frightening in its own right. These episodes of extreme anxiety are marked by physical symptoms such as dizziness, numbness, tingling, breathlessness, heart palpitations, sweating, and unreality. They are called panic attacks, and panic disorder is an anxiety condition characterized by recurrent panic attacks. Each of the symptoms of a panic attack makes sense. The physical symptoms are either a direct effect of anxiety (e.g., rapid heart rate, rapid breathing, sweating) or a secondary effect of other symptomatic responses (e.g., rapid breathing can rapidly lead to feelings of dizziness and unreality). These symptoms are commonplace at times of fear and are a natural reaction to danger. In an actual dangerous situation (for example, being threatened by another person), attention is focused on the actual threat rather than on these symptoms. However, if these anxiety symptoms occur out of the blue, they can become a focus of attention in their own right.

In panic disorder, it is not uncommon for individuals to interpret these symptoms as a sign of one or more of the following:

- Impending death (*Am I having a heart attack?; Am I having a stroke?; I am going to die!*)
- Impending loss of control (*I will faint; I am going to have to run out of the room; I can't find my way out or take care of the kids*)
- Impending humiliation (*They are going to notice my symptoms and I will be humiliated; They will think I am crazy; They will think I am a fool*)

These interpretations are of course among the most frightening thoughts a person can have. If believed, these thoughts should motivate the very anxiety reactions that are feared. This is the essence of panic disorder. It is a disorder characterized by the fear of anxiety sensations—the fear of fear itself!

Panic disorder, with or without the avoidance of feared situations (agoraphobia), occurs in about 3% of adults. Panic attacks themselves are much more common, but the full disorder is diagnosed only when the panic attacks are a source of concern themselves. In the full disorder, having panic attacks several times a week is common. Individuals with panic disorder become so concerned about the possibility of having these attacks that they may avoid a wide variety of situations where these attacks might occur (agoraphobia). Avoided situations frequently include those where escape may be difficult (should a panic attack occur)—for example, being on a bus, on a bridge, in a long line, in a crowded room, on the subway, driving far from home, in a movie theater, and in a shopping mall.

Panic disorder frequently begins after a period of stress, but what appears to put people at risk for the disorder is the tendency to fear anxiety-related sensations. In addition, once panic disorder develops, it both sensitizes people toward and intensifies this fear of symptoms.

Fears of symptoms can take the usual "what if" form that characterizes other anxiety-provoking thoughts, such as:

- *What if other people notice?*
- *What if I have a heart attack?*
- *What if I fall down?*
- *What if it gets worse, I lose control, and I start to scream?*
- *What if I go crazy?*
- *What if I have a stroke?*

After initial attacks, a self-perpetuating pattern can develop to maintain and worsen the panic attacks. Becoming overly focused on anxiety sensations (*I hope it does not happen now; is my heart beating fast yet?*), memories of past attacks (*Last time was horrible! I hope that does not happen again*), and fears of future attacks (*I am starting to lose control; it could be worse than ever*) all combine to amplify initial signs of anxiety into a full panic attack. With repeated panic attacks, your body may directly start to respond to signs of arousal (rapid heart rate, sweating, dizziness, etc.) by firing what we call the "alarm reaction."

Over time, individuals with panic disorder can become sensitized to these sensations regardless of their source. For example, coffee and exercise produce only mild sensations similar to anxiety (increased heart rate, sweating, and trembling), but because these sensations are linked to the fears of panic attacks, individuals with panic disorder may come to fear these natural sensations and avoid coffee, exercise, and other events that produce even mild symptoms. A result is that individuals with panic disorder always feel on alert for the possibility of another panic attack; they are over-vigilant to how their body is feeling (autonomic arousal) and ready to tense up and avoid or control these sensations should they emerge. This essential pattern underlying panic disorder is summarized in Figure 10.2.

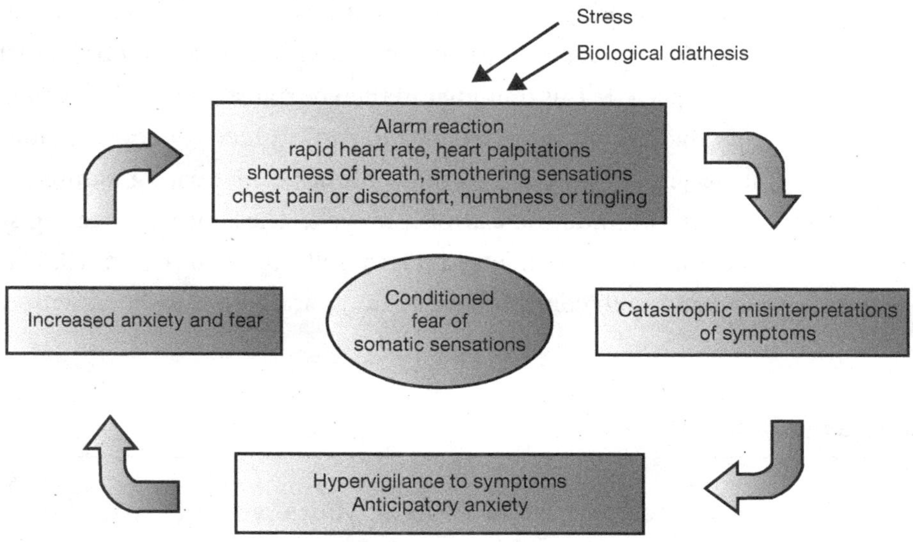

Figure 10.2

Cognitive-Behavioral Model of Panic Disorder

One of the most effective treatments for panic disorder is cognitive-behavioral therapy (CBT). Reviewing your symptoms with your therapist can help confirm whether you have a diagnosis of panic disorder, and if you do, you will want to learn about the disorder and its treatment. The core elements of CBT for panic disorder include information about the disorder, help in eliminating the power of "what if" thoughts, and exposure to the feared sensations associated with anxiety and panic. As noted, a variety of these sensations can be induced by vigorous exercise, and, as such, exercise can be used as part of treatment for panic disorder.

With vigorous exercise, you can learn to eliminate fears of anxiety sensations by taking charge and becoming comfortable with these natural sensations of your body at work. Vigorous exercise will naturally produce any of a number of odd sensations, such as:

- Rapid heart rate or a "pounding" heart
- Rapid breathing
- A feeling of a heavy chest (from breathing hard)
- Heavy legs
- Sweating
- Dizziness or light-headedness
- Dry mouth or throat
- Numb hands (while running)

The goal of bringing on these sensations (all sensations of autonomic arousal) is to let yourself become comfortable with them and embrace them as natural and expected. This training can then be transferred back to similar sensations that may arise due to anxiety and panic. Once you learn to undo the fear of these sensations, you can undo the self-perpetuating nature of panic. That is, you can undo the fear-of-fear cycle. The shift from fearing symptoms to becoming comfortable with them is illustrated in Figure 10.3. The goal is to do nothing to control the sensations, and rather to "relax with" them.

Applying Exercise to Panic Disorder

As you increase the intensity of your exercise (as your fitness increases), part of the goal will be to exercise vigorously enough to produce bodily

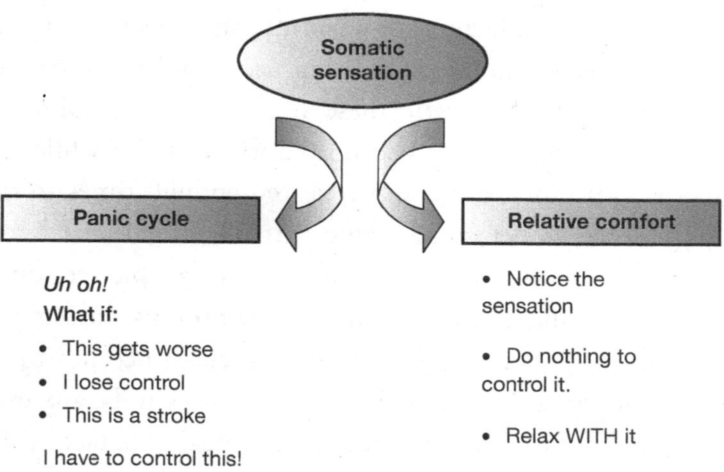

Figure 10.3

Reacting Differently to Panic Sensations

sensations similar to those you experience during a panic attack. Prior to and during this vigorous exercise, you will want to:

1. Remind yourself of what sensations you are going to feel so that there are no surprises (e.g., rapid breathing, rapid heart rate, and sweating are normal reactions to vigorous exercise).
2. Complete the exercise, fully expecting to experience these sensations.
3. Notice the sensations and see how comfortable you can get exercising *while having the sensations.*

Then, after you complete the exercise, try not to be waiting for the sensations to go away. Just become good at tolerating them. Remind yourself that it does not matter how long they last because they are not dangerous (your physician has approved your exercise); therefore, you don't have to get rid of these sensations.

Your therapist may play an active role in using exercise in this way—as part of formal "exposure therapy" directed at the feared sensations that underlie panic disorder. For exposure therapy, therapists provide organized and step-by-step experiences getting used to feared situations and sensations. Therapists tend to start this work by reviewing what the exposure experience will be like. In the case of using exercise in exposure therapy, this means the review of some of the natural sensations to be experienced during exercise (e.g., rapid heart rate; rapid breathing;

sweaty skin; feelings of warmth; some breathlessness; tired, sore, or odd feelings in the muscles being used) and some preparation for the notion of *relaxing with* these symptoms (i.e., doing nothing to manage these symptoms, just calmly noticing them while you continue to exercise). Then exercise is repeated enough times so that you can have a chance to get comfortable with or even bored by these symptoms—these symptoms are simply the way people feel during exercise. After developing comfort with these symptoms during exercise, your therapist may then help you apply this sense of comfort to anxiety symptoms more broadly. When this is done successfully, anxiety does not progress into panic, and the regular panic attacks characteristic of panic disorder are shut down.

Increasing Your Target Heart Rate

To help treat panic disorder, exercise intensity will have to be high enough to bring on the bodily sensations that you experience during a panic attack. For this purpose, you may want to increase the target heart range for your exercise sessions to the middle or high range (80–85% HR_{max}) of vigorous-intensity exercise. If you chose to experiment with increasing your heart rate during your workouts, fill out Worksheet 10.1: Your Exercise Prescription for Targeting Panic. Worksheets can be found at the end of this chapter or can be accessed by searching for this book's title on the Oxford Academic platform, at academic.oup.com. A completed example of this worksheet is provided in Figure 10.4.

Week	Exercise intensity	Exercise duration	Exercise frequency
5	75% of HR_{max}	20 minutes	3 times per week
6	80% of HR_{max}	20 minutes	3 times per week
7	85% of HR_{max}	20–25 minutes	3–4 times per week
8	85% of HR_{max}	25–30 minutes	3–5 times per week

Figure 10.4

Example of a Completed Worksheet 10.1: Your Exercise Prescription for Targeting Panic

To help you with the task of becoming comfortable with intense bodily sensations, you may want to keep a log of your experiences during vigorous exercise. Worksheet 10.2: Exercise Practice Log for Panic-Related Concerns is designed to draw your attention to the sensations you experience during exercise and help you become confident that they are safe. On the worksheet, you are asked to record the sensations, rate their intensity on a 0-to-100 scale, and rate whether the experience of anxiety was associated with anxiety on the same scale. Then you are asked to examine whether the symptoms had any true negative consequences for you relative to your fears of these sensations. Bring your completed logs for review with your therapist to help you consolidate some of the gains you are achieving from exercise.

Applying What You Learned to Your Anxiety and Panic

Worksheet 10.2 is designed to help you approach your panic symptoms in a new way, based on your experiences with exercise sensations. As you repeat your exercise sessions (using a new log each time), notice how you are getting more comfortable with the sensations you induce with vigorous exercise. Also notice how you are carrying your shoulders during exercise. If you are running, are you able to relax your shoulders and arms? This is part of the skill of relaxing with anxiety-like sensations: letting the sensations occur but doing nothing to manage them and letting your shoulders and arms relax. As you notice this ability during your run (or other exercise), think how you can apply this new ability (of not being pushed around by anxiety-like sensations) to the times when you get anxious or panicky. Indeed, the next time you feel anxious at work or at home, coach yourself to apply your running skill—for example, *I can relax with anxiety-like body sensations when I run; let me apply that same skill now. I am going to practice accepting my feeling of anxiety and still be relatively comfortable in my body.* Work with your therapist to help you extend these gains and end regular anxiety and panic cycles.

Worksheet 10.1: Your Exercise Prescription for Targeting Panic

Please select the exercise intensity, duration, and frequency for your workouts so that this week can help you create greater comfort with the bodily sensations of autonomic arousal.

Week	Exercise intensity	Exercise duration	Exercise frequency

Worksheet 10.2: Exercise Practice Log for Panic-Related Concerns

Date of exercise: _________

What exercise did you do?

____

What sensations did you experience during your exercise?

____

____

How intense were the sensations during your workout (0–100)?

Beginning:

Halfway:

Toward the end:

What was your anxiety level throughout the session (0–100)?

Beginning:

Halfway:

Toward the end:

What were the consequences of the sensations that you experienced?

____

____

How did these consequences differ from the fears you had of these sensations due to your panic disorder?

____

____

What do you want to tell yourself about these sensations now?

____

____

____

GOALS

- To understand how exercise can aid cognition
- To look at specific bouts of exercise for cognition
- To consider exercise as a prevention for cognitive decline

OVERVIEW

Exercise offers some dramatic benefits to brain health. This chapter provides you with information on the nature of these benefits and how you might use exercise to improve your memory, attention, and general cognition.

Exercise, BDNF, and Your Brain

In Chapter 2, we introduced you to a brain-maintenance and memory molecule called BDNF (brain-derived neurotrophic factor) and let you know that exercise enhances BDNF activity in your brain. This is really good news because BDNF has a few crucial functions. BDNF supports your brain's functioning overall and helps your brain cells (neurons) grow and thrive. BDNF is also involved in the way the brain forms memories, helping these memories be available for guiding your ongoing functioning, including the ability to hold your attention on and think about multiple items/concepts (in other words, your working memory). Exercise and

BDNF are good for helping maintain or improve some of the thinking processes we use every day.

How does exercise do this? As noted in Chapter 2 (do you remember?), if we think about BDNF in terms of a Miracle-Gro® metaphor, just as Miracle-Gro® helps plants thrive, each session of exercise is metaphorically similar to pouring Miracle-Gro® BDNF over the brain. You can expect some short-lived cognitive benefits from each workout—meaning that you can use exercise to refresh your cognition for the period of time following a workout. For example, if you are having a stressful day and have some problems to solve, think of using exercise to give yourself a cognitive boost. If you are a student and studying for a test, think of using exercise to help lock in the material you studied. Moderate exercise works best in these situations; save the high-intensity exercise for when you are not preparing for a test or solving a work problem.

There are also stronger BDNF benefits of exercise when you continue a program of exercise. That is, when you work out regularly, more metaphorical Miracle-Gro® is poured over the brain with each bout of exercise. Longer-term programs of exercise (for example, regular walking for 40 minutes four times a week) help improve mild cognitive impairments associated with aging and have shown promise for slowing the decline associated with specific brain diseases like Alzheimer's disease or Parkinson's disease. If you are at risk for one of these diseases, we strongly recommend that you get clearance from your physician and start a regular program of exercise, following the guidance provided throughout this workbook.

There are additional psychiatric conditions involving cognitive impairments that have also shown clear benefit from exercise. For example, the cognitive deficits associated with depression improve with a program of exercise, effectively doubling the sort of improvement you can expect when exercising to treat depression (both mood and cognitive benefits). Exercise also helps the cognitive impairment seen in disorders like schizophrenia, where thinking impairments appear to be at the heart of the disorder. Regular exercise has been shown to reduce these cognitive impairments.

How Do You Want to Use Exercise for Cognition?

Because there are both short- and long-term benefits from exercise for cognition, consider which of these benefits you and your therapist might want to apply. For example, in addition to providing you with a refresh in brain power for work or school, you could try exercising before your therapy session. Potential benefits of this approach include:

- You may go into the therapy session more relaxed and in a better mood—a very helpful effect if you are planning to talk about difficult topics.
- Given that you likely were sweating and had a high heart rate during exercise, it is less likely that feelings of anxiety will be as bothersome during the session.
- The BDNF activity following a combined exercise and therapy session appears to make it more likely that you will retain learning from your therapy session. This may be particularly useful for exposure therapy, where you are actively trying to relearn a sense of safety around situations or events that have frightened you.

These three benefits of a bout of exercise before a therapy session—better mood, less anxiety reactivity, and enhanced memory—may make it easier to face your fears and retain your learning of safety from the session. Such work can be coordinated with your therapist to get the best out of your planned therapy.

If, however, you are interested in the long-term benefits of exercise for cognition—for example, you want to reduce some of the cognitive slowing that happens with age or you are at risk for the loss of cognitive abilities due to a condition like Alzheimer's disease—then you will want to work toward starting and maintaining a longer-term program of exercise. As discussed throughout this workbook, and specifically in the final chapter (Chapter 14), maintaining a longer-term program of exercise will require a focus on finding joy in your workouts and being open to changing up your exercise enough to keep it interesting. In doing so, do not forget the value of a support team—those individuals who will remind you of your motivations for exercise and, hopefully, will join you in your exercise program. If needed, take a fresh look at Worksheet 1.3: Selecting Members of Your Support Team. If you give the gift of exercise to others, know that they can also expect to get the mood and cognitive benefits that you are pursuing.

And as a final note, let's not leave your pets out of these considerations. Walking or running with your dog can be a particular joy, and there is even research indicating your dog will get cognitive benefits from regular exercise.

Exercise for Psychological Resilience

- To introduce the concept of psychological resilience
- To understand how exercise can help with resilience
- To expand your understanding of a mind/body balance
- To develop an Exercise+ strategy for promoting mindfulness
- To extend your use of psychological resilience

An advisory committee to the U.S. Department of Health and Human Services labeled exercise as a " 'best buy' for public health." Throughout the early chapters of this workbook, you read about the meaning of this statement: In addition to its physical benefits, exercise has broad benefits for improving mood, reducing anxiety, and enhancing cognition. Given these benefits, it should come as no surprise that exercise is also known to enhance psychological resilience—the ability to recover ("bounce back") from stress and adversity.

Multiple studies show that regular exercise protects against negative emotional responses to stress, protects against how reactive the body is to stress (for example, the degree to which your body releases stress hormones), and protects against burnout from stressful school or work environments. Regular exercise naturally increases resilience, and this chapter enhances that training.

There is no bad time to think about starting an exercise-for-resilience program. Your therapist might suggest that you read this chapter early in your treatment program to add to other treatment efforts, trying to achieve broader benefits than you might get by psychotherapy or medication treatment alone. Or your therapist may ask you to read this chapter as part of relapse-prevention efforts. Relapse prevention refers to those procedures used to help keep you well after most of your core symptoms—for instance, your depression or anxiety—have resolved. The goal of relapse prevention is to take you further toward feelings of well-being and to provide additional protections against factors that may place you at risk for relapse—factors like stress.

In applying exercise to relapse prevention, pay attention to the benefits of exercise, considerations for dose and intensity, and the management of barriers to exercise as discussed in the first six chapters of this workbook. Then, once your exercise program is established, we would like you to think about three specific exercise-for-resilience considerations: mind–body balance, mindful exercise, and expanding your resilience to life situations.

Mind/Body Balance

Exercising your body to benefit your mind and mood is a strategy to achieve mind/body balance. An exercise-for-resilience program is an extension of this focus on a mind/body balance as summarized by a simple prescription: *Seek a balance between useful action and useful rest, especially at times of stress.* What does this mean? Working to maintain at least 7 hours of sleep a night during periods of enhanced stress helps your mind erase some of the emotional burden of stress, so that the stress does not get worse over a difficult week. Also, doubling down on your commitment to regular exercise during a stressful week is important, particularly given the many exercise-derailing thoughts that come at a time of stress:

- *Ugh, I feel tired. Why would I work out now?*
- *I need a break from doing anything because I feel so stressed.*
- *Why work out now when I already feel wrung-out from the day?*

Exercise 12.1: List of Common Reactions to Stress

When stressed or upset during a difficult week, do you . . .

- Have a few (alcoholic) drinks
- Eat too much ice cream
- Search online for a "comfort" purchase
- Use cannabis
- Stay up late watching mindless television
- Eat comfort food
- Get lost in Facebook or Instagram
- Smoke a cigarette

A moderate workout may be the very thing you need to feel recovered from a stressful day. But be assured that it is OK to have lighter workouts when feeling stressed or fatigued. This is part of mind–body balance as well—learning to not push yourself too hard during periods of stress. Easy workouts during an especially stressful week will still give your body what it needs to provide stress resilience. Consider this helpful thought, "The weight of stress may very well be less after a workout."

Stressful weeks are also a time to consider some of the many things people do that are opposite to the core mind/body advice to *seek a balance between useful action and useful rest, especially at times of stress.* Exercise 12.1 provides a list of common reactions to stress.

Each of these options, if selected as a regular response to stress, can worsen mood and lead to chronic cycles of distress. On the other hand, Exercise 12.2 lists some of the strategies to cope with stress that follow the recommendation to *seek a balance between useful action and useful rest, especially at times of stress.*

Exercising at a time of stress is simply a strategy to respect the mind/body connection and to use the body in service of both your mind and mood. In doing so, you can be assured that you are building an excellent habit for the future (maintaining your exercise program despite having a low or anxious mood) and continuing to train your body to be less reactive to stress to provide yourself with greater well-being in the future.

Exercise+: Adding Mindfulness to Exercise

As introduced in Chapter 3 of this workbook, Exercise+ is a strategy of making exercise more interesting by adding something to it. For example, in Chapter 3 we discussed adding an audiobook to exercise. By allowing yourself to listen to that (hopefully exciting) book only during exercise, a desire to listen to the book should naturally pull you toward exercise. With this method, you do not have to push yourself to exercise; you need only restrict the audiobook to your exercise sessions.

In this chapter, we discuss the use of mindfulness as an Exercise+ strategy. Unlike the audiobook example, mindfulness is not to be done exclusively during exercise, but is instead done to make exercise more rewarding and to deepen any mindfulness practice you may have as part of a therapy program, yoga, or perhaps online training. Mindfulness is itself a strategy for psychological resilience, and so adding it to your exercise-for-resilience program has the potential to enhance your resilience abilities nicely.

There are two key features of mindfulness that we would like you to rehearse during exercise: (1) present-focused attention and (2) an open and accepting attitude toward the objects of your attention. Concerning attention, a present focus for exercise means directing your attention to the many aspects of current experience (what is happening right now) instead of past or future experience. When it comes to a run, for example, it would mean refocusing attention on the current experience of the run rather than thinking about the distance left or the time remaining in the workout. It also involves appreciating the wealth of current experience you have during the workout, such as the physical sensations, thoughts, feelings, and the sensory stimulation that occurs during a run: the cool crispness of the air, the sounds of your foot strikes on the sandy soil, feeling the breeze more on the left side of your body than the right, the color of the tree ahead of you as silhouetted against the evening sky. There is a lot going on, and much to appreciate if you allow your attention to flow through these experiences. This is the first step of mindfulness: to notice the topics of your current focus and to expand this focus to include a broader range of current experience.

All too often, though, attention during exercise may become stuck on one channel (e.g., "my left knee hurts"), and the wealth of the exercise experience may be lost. To mindfully run means to remind yourself to let your attention roam without pushing anything out of your experience but also not getting stuck on any one thing. You may notice that your left knee hurts *and* be able to appreciate the look of the tree against the evening sky *and* notice the breeze cooling your skin more on the left side than the right side of your body. The "and" is important: It reflects your ability to shift and hold your attention among many channels at once, appreciating whatever input is there.

The word "appreciate" brings us to the second facet of mindfulness we want you to practice during exercise: being open to your present experiences. This component of mindfulness involves accepting the object of your attention without judging. When it comes to noticing the breeze on your skin, the goal is to feel it without categorizing it as perhaps too warm or too cold or too breezy or not breezy enough. Judgments are verbal categorizations of current experience, and with such judgments the world falls into categories of good or bad, acceptable or unacceptable. For example:

- *My run is too slow.*
- *I am too tired.*
- *I am lousy at running.*
- *I am sweating too much.*

To run more mindfully, the key is to treat a judgment as an experience. When faced by a judging thought like, "I am a lousy runner," the shift to observing this thought takes the form, "I am having the thought that I am lousy at running." The thought is just one more aspect of experience that can be attended to or not.

Let's take another common thought that occurs during running: "I want my run to be over now." To treat this thought as an experience, add the phrase "I am having the thought that . . ." so that the thought becomes, "I am having the thought that I want my run to be over now." Doing this can make the thought feel less pressing and more like the many other experiences you are having at the moment, so that it is easier to let your experiences flow from this one thought to those other aspects of your

Exercise 12.3: Six Steps to a More Mindful Exercise

During ongoing exercise, try the following:

Step 1. Notice where your attention is going—whether you are in the moment or thinking about the past or future—and notice which specific aspects of your current experience are capturing your attention.

Step 2. Take a deep breath and let it out, and check your facial expression: Relax your face and let yourself have a half-smile in preparation for your mindful experience.

Step 3. Practice letting your attention float through aspects of your current experience. Try to have your attention flow through at least two aspects of your sensory experience (feelings on your skin), two aspects of your auditory experience (sounds you hear), and two aspects of your visual experience (e.g., colors you see).

Step 4. As you continue your exercise and notice your attention being caught by a particular event, sensation, or thought, note your attention to this experience and then add an "and," gently shifting your attention to a different sensation or aspect of your current experience.

Step 5. If you notice that a particular thought is dominating your attention, reframe your thought as an observation: "I am having the thought that . . ." and then again add an "and," gently shifting your attention to a different sensation or aspect of your current experience.

Step 6. Repeat Steps 1 through 5, and appreciate the experience.

current experience (e.g., your shoes striking the sandy soil; the tree framed by the evening sky).

Practicing mindful attention during exercising can have the direct benefit of making your run more enjoyable and relaxing. It also has the secondary effect of building stronger mindfulness skills. That is, you may have learned (or now may be curious to learn) mindfulness skills when sitting silently as part of yoga or as part of instruction from a therapist or web-based video. But taking mindfulness out into the world, while you are acting, can be thought of as the next-level mindfulness. You don't have to be silent or sitting, and you can bring mindfulness into any moment you choose in your life. This is a benefit of practicing Exercise+ using mindfulness.

Tips for starting your Exercise+ mindfulness program are provided in Exercise 12.3.

Extending Your Resilience

In addition to boosting your mood, we would like to remind you of the ways in which exercise can increase your comfort with sensations of anxiety. As discussed in Chapter 10, regular exercise, particularly more vigorous exercise, can help you get used to (more comfortable with) the emotional and physical experience of anxiety. This occurs because exercise regularly exposes you to so many of these sensations—rapid heart rate, rapid breathing, sweating, breathlessness, facial flushing, heavy legs, etc.—and your ability to persist enjoyably (e.g., continue your run, and perhaps even continue your run mindfully while having these sensations) is excellent training for being able to react differently to anxiety in all sorts of situations.

It is helpful to occasionally check in with yourself to see if this is true. For example, the next time you have a difficult work meeting, or a difficult interaction with a relative, see if you are able to stay calmer even though your body might be reacting with anxiety or anger. Are you able to be a better problem-solver in this situation because you are not distracted or distressed by your body's reaction? Are you better able to stay in the game without avoidance—showing up at a difficult meeting and being the one to speak up about an issue? These are important features of resilience. Exercise both decreases your body's reaction to stress and can increase your comfort with the stressful bodily reactions you do have. When you discover these benefits, lean into them and thank your runs, bike rides, or swims for this benefit to your stress management.

It is also useful to consider some of the *physical* resilience that is provided by regular exercise. Because your body will adapt to what you demand of it physically, you may now have new opportunities for activities. Greater fitness from an exercise program that started with walking and then progressed to running may lead you to feel good about joining a volleyball team, or more vigorously playing with the kids, or hiking to the top of the mountain with friends. Greater comfort with swimming as part of your exercise program may lead you to consider snorkeling, windsurfing, or scuba diving while on vacation. This is part of the physical resilience that an exercise program offers—it can open doors to a broader range of values-based activities and make those activities more achievable due to improved fitness.

CHAPTER 13 — Smoking Cessation and Other Habit Control

GOALS

- To identify the process of quitting smoking and smoking withdrawal symptoms
- To understand how exercise can help with withdrawal symptoms
- To consider the resources you need for a successful quit attempt
- To develop your quit plan
- To use exercise for smoking cessation success
- To think about other unhealthy habits to target

OVERVIEW

Because exercise can enhance resilience for some of the factors that can derail habit change, exercise can be used to increase the success of difficult tasks like quitting smoking. In this chapter we provide information about planning a quit attempt and tell you how an exercise program can help make that attempt more successful.

Introduction

Quitting smoking is an excellent way to benefit your health and extend your life, and to increase the health of those around you. And by quitting smoking you are joining the majority of adults in the United States: Currently only 1 out of 8 men and 1 out of 10 women are smokers.

We know that quitting smoking is hard. It is hard because nicotine is highly addictive and stopping smoking means that you will go through a period of time when you are challenged by withdrawal sensations on your path to being free of smoking. Quitting is also hard because, for most smokers, smoking is part of a daily routine that provides lots of reminders to smoke, and it is common to have increased cravings to smoke when confronted by a variety of situations or emotional states associated with smoking.

Why Does Exercise Help Smoking Cessation?

As you know from reading earlier chapters in this workbook, regular exercise improves mood, reduces anxiety, reduces the degree to which anxiety-related symptoms are bothersome, improves cognition, and improves sleep. Now let's consider the symptoms of nicotine withdrawal that emerge soon after quitting: depressed mood, irritability, anxiety, restlessness, difficulty concentrating, and insomnia. Sound familiar? There is a very tight match between symptoms of withdrawal and some of the effects of regular exercise. This is why exercise helps with smoking cessation. Exercise appears to reduce sensitivity to the withdrawal sensations and the sad, anxious, or irritable moods that accompany a quit attempt, so that these sensations and moods do not push people back to smoking. In other words, regular exercise offers a well-designed program for smoking cessation, helping you become resilient to some of the classic causes of smoking relapse.

It is also important to consider other tools that can help with stopping smoking: social support, medication, and skills for coping with craving. Social support is important for any change effort: Valued friends or family members can remind you of your goals and help you through the tough periods of behavior change. Medications like nicotine replacement therapy (nicotine in lozenges, gums, or patches), varenicline, or bupropion have a range of effects that resemble those of regular exercise: They can reduce the degree of craving, withdrawal sensations, and mood changes that accompany a quit attempt. Similarly, counseling programs for smoking cessation devote effort to help smokers develop a plan for how to react differently (e.g., distraction, deep breathing) to cues for smoking, including cravings driven by these cues and withdrawal sensations.

It has never been easier to access these smoking cessation treatment strategies. The Centers for Disease Control and Prevention (CDC) has a number of programs to provide information and planning for your quit attempt. Information on smoking cessation challenges and treatment strategies is available through their comprehensive website (https://www.cdc.gov/tobacco/campaign/tips/quit-smoking/index.html), with specific help provided as part of a telephone quit hotline (1-800-784-8669). You can also download their QuitStart App from Google Play or the Apple Store.

Motivational information for quitting smoking is provided by the TIPS Program, also from the CDC. This video-based program lets you hear frank talk from ex-smokers who wish they had quit smoking earlier. They are adults who are living with some of the long-term health effects from smoking or exposure to secondhand smoke (breathing smoke from others). There are also videos from family members who take care of loved ones who have disease or disability from smoking. This information is available at https://www.cdc.gov/tobacco/campaign/tips/index.html.

What About Vaping?

All of the information in this chapter can be applied to vaping as well as smoking, including being ready for withdrawal sensations, being ready for cues to vape, and learning how to use exercise to help your quitting program succeed.

How to Start an Exercise for Smoking Cessation Program

Most of the information you need for an exercise for smoking cessation program can be found in the previous chapters of this workbook. In many ways, exercise for stopping smoking represents the combination of exercise for mood (Chapter 8) and exercise for anxiety-related sensations (Chapter 10), with the goal of eliminating these vulnerabilities to smoking relapse (mood and sensitivity to anxiety-related sensations).

We always encourage you to modify your exercise program to provide the best fit for your lifestyle and interests, but the prototypic exercise for a smoking cessation program includes the following elements:

1. Because smoking increases your cardiovascular health risks, seek approval from your physician for your program of exercise.
2. Start your exercise program at least 5 weeks before your smoking quit date.

3. In the 2 weeks before your quit attempt, progress your aerobic exercise (e.g., rapid walking, biking, running, swimming) to vigorous intensity. As you may recall from Chapter 5, vigorous-intensity exercise is defined by heart rate ranges between 77% and 93% of your HR_{max}. Use the formula provided below to determine your target heart rate:

Vigorous-intensity exercise

77% to 93% × (220 − your age) =_______ to_______%

4. For your smoking cessation program, try to do 75 minutes of exercise in your target heart rate zone each week, divided across two or three exercise sessions.

How to Create a Smoking Cessation "Quit Plan"

To help you successfully quit smoking, it is important to go into your quit attempt with a clear plan that includes your motivations to quit, your support team, your use of medication if desired, and your plan for your period of cravings. In the sections below we describe each of these elements of a quit plan and then provide you with Worksheet 13.1: Individualized Quite Plan for Smoking to formalize this planning. You can also complete similar quit planning online through https://smokefree.gov/build-your-quit-plan.

Clear Motivations for Change

When changing any well-ingrained behavior, it makes good sense to get your motivations really clear. Clear motivations are useful at the outset of planning to quit smoking to help you consider the range of tools you want to use to make your quit attempt a success. Clear motivations are also useful for the challenging points you will face after your quit date, when—perhaps 10 days after quitting smoking, after a stressful day—you have the thought, "Maybe I could have just one."

Common reasons for stopping smoking include the following:

- To improve your health (e.g., reduction in heart attack or cancer risk)
- To improve the health of your family (from secondhand smoke)
- To feel more in control (not dependent on nicotine to feel OK)
- To save money (yearly cost: $ per pack × packs per week × 52 weeks in a year)
- To set a good example (for family or friends)
- For your family and friends who don't like being around smoke
- Because your doctor recommended it
- To look better and to not smell like smoke
- To eliminate the aggravation of trying to find a place to smoke
- Because you are tired of the daily cycles of craving

Consider these reasons and see if you have unique ones of your own. On Worksheet 13.1, you will be asked to list your own top-three reasons.

Your Stop-Smoking Team

It will also be important for you to consider who is going to be on your support team for smoking cessation. You want these people to want the best health for you and to be prepared to remind you of your cessation goals and commend you for your efforts. These are also the people who may join you in nonsmoking situations (e.g., going to a movie) to help you through a rough period of craving. We like the act of announcing your quit date to your team—that announcement will help you keep your intentions to quit active.

Medication Use for Quit Success

Medications can also be used to help you with your quit attempt. In general, these medications work by reducing both the degree of craving and withdrawal sensations. One medication strategy is to replace the nicotine in tobacco products with nicotine provided in patches, gum, or lozenges. These nicotine replacement therapies (NRTs) are the most commonly used quit-smoking medications. By replacing the nicotine that was in your tobacco, these medications prevent the stronger withdrawal sensations so that you can give up the behavioral habit of smoking separately from having to cope with the withdrawal symptoms. Then, over time, as you feel more secure in your quit attempt, you taper down your use of the NRT. NRT is routinely considered a safe option to aid smoking cessation, except for higher-risk groups such as pregnant women or teens. Dosing information is provided on the package insert, and typically the NRT dose is matched to the amount you are smoking and is started before the quit attempt. You can buy NRTs without a prescription (they are over-the-counter medications), and in many locations you can use state programs to get them for free. (Check your local smoking cessation website.) Some people get side effects from NRTs, and the package insert has information on coping with these side effects.

Other common medication options include varenicline and bupropion. Both of these medications are available by prescription and will require you to visit your physician to discuss their pros and cons and whether they are right for you. Used correctly, these medications in conjunction with your exercise program can greatly increase your likelihood of quitting smoking for good. Like NRT, the most common recommendation is to start the medication and get on a stable dose for a period of time before your quit date.

Preparing for Smoking Triggers

Before your quit date, it is also important for you to understand the situational and emotional triggers you have for smoking. Common triggers are listed in Table 13.1.

Think about your triggers and add them to the appropriate section of Worksheet 13.1. (Worksheets can be found at the end of this chapter or can be accessed by searching for this book's title on the Oxford Academic platform, at academic.oup.com.)

The worksheet also provides you with a list of coping responses for getting through a rough period of craving without having a smoke. In general, these strategies include things that are stimulating to your mouth and hands to replace the feel of having a cigarette or vape pen (e.g., chewing gum, fiddling with a pencil, chewing a handy crunchy snack like carrots), calming distractions (deep breathing, drinking ice water), and moving yourself to a nonsmoking situation (e.g., a gym, movie theater, restaurant, or library). In addition, using exercise, or even a reminder of your exercise

<u>Situational cues for smoking</u>

- ☐ After waking up
- ☐ Before going to bed
- ☐ Driving
- ☐ When having an alcoholic drink
- ☐ When drinking coffee
- ☐ When you want to concentrate
- ☐ Mid-morning
- ☐ After work
- ☐ After sex

<u>Emotional cues for smoking</u>

- ☐ When you feel sad
- ☐ When you feel stressed or anxious
- ☐ When you feel tired
- ☐ When you feel frustrated
- ☐ When you want to relax
- ☐ When you feel irritated

program (doing 10 sit-ups, 10 jumping jacks, etc.), can help stave off a period of craving and remind yourself of the program of mood and resilience boost you are on with exercise. Before your quit date, further planning and rehearsal of skills for smoking cessation can be provided by a "practice-quit" program that is designed to use daily challenges to help you build your skills for understanding smoking triggers and managing cravings.

Preparing Your Quit Plan Worksheet

Considering the elements of a quit plan, go ahead and fill out Worksheet 13.1. Note that you can modify this worksheet at any point during your smoking cessation journey, changing your coping strategies as you learn more about the situations and emotions that affect your cravings for smoking. If you prefer an online quit plan, remember you can use resources provided by the federal government at https://smokefree.gov/build-your-quit-plan.

A Lapse Is Not a Relapse

If you do happen to have a smoke after your quit date, we want you to remember that a lapse (having a "slip") is not a relapse (a return to regular smoking patterns). Slips are relatively common, so it pays not to be too hard on yourself. Instead we would like you to learn from the slip: Try to figure out what happened so that your urges beat out your motivations to stop smoking. Are there triggers to smoke that you need to avoid for a while, or do you need to rehearse new ways in which to cope with them? Have you discussed the slip with your quit team? Are there ways you can kick up your exercise plan to both underscore your level of healthful fitness and increase your emotional resilience? Do you need to make any revisions to your quit plan? Consider answers to these questions and then plan to restart quitting as soon as you can—today or tomorrow.

Applying Exercise to Other Habit Control

The methods described above—use of exercise to increase emotional resilience combined with a broader plan to address unhealthful habits with multiple strategies and social support—can also be applied to other habits you would like to control. Many other habits have patterns keeping them going that are similar to smoking: driven by strong urges and the desire to avoid negative emotional states like withdrawal. Even a bad habit like overusing the internet for procrastination (also called "cyberloafing" or "internet addiction") seems to be driven, in part, by intolerance of negative emotions. That is, for many people, over-clicking online is a form of self-soothing when other important responsibilities are calling but are too emotionally uncomfortable to address. This means that you can use your exercise program to enhance your emotional resilience (creating better mood and greater tolerance to negative bodily and emotional sensations while also rehearsing useful action) and then apply this ability to your habit change goals. As we recommend for smoking, prior to your change attempt we would like you to think through your motivations, your support team, high-risk situations and emotions that might derail your behavioral change goals, and your coping plans for these high-risk events. You can use Worksheet 13.2: Your Habit Change Plan to help create a plan to work on other habits you would like to address.

Worksheet 13.1: Individualized Quit Plan for Smoking

Your top three reasons for quitting smoking are:

1.

2.

3.

When you feel an urge to have a smoke, you want to remind yourself that (encouragements to get past a smoking urge):

1.

2.

3.

Your quit-smoking team (people who will be supportive of a quit attempt and who would be there to help you get past a period of strong smoking cravings):

1.

2.

3.

Quit-smoking medications you might consider include:

- ☐ NRT (nicotine replacement patches, gum, or lozenges; available over the counter)
- ☐ Varenicline (requires prescription)
- ☐ Bupropion (requires prescription)
- ☐ No medication

Your top cues for smoking:

Situational	Emotional
1.	1.
2.	2.
3.	3.
4.	4.

Strategies to use when cravings strike:

- ☐ Chew gum
- ☐ Place a toothpick, straw, or cinnamon stick in your mouth
- ☐ Eat hard candy or lollipops
- ☐ Eat carrot sticks
- ☐ Use a squeeze ball
- ☐ Fiddle with a pencil
- ☐ Drink a glass of cold water
- ☐ Complete a breathing exercise
- ☐ Jog in place briefly (or do jumping jacks)
- ☐ Do 10 push-ups
- ☐ Call a friend
- ☐ Engage with your smartphone
- ☐ Move out of a high-risk situation
- ☐ Go to a movie (or other nonsmoking situation)
- ☐ Review your quit-smoking motivations

Your quit date (the date you select for starting a smoke-free future) is: __________

Prior to your quit date you should:

- ☐ Rid your home, workplace, and car of cigarettes, vapes, lighters, ashtrays, etc.
- ☐ Wash clothes and other items that smell of tobacco smoke.
- ☐ Inform your quit team of your quit date.
- ☐ Feel really good about your plan to make yourself smoke-free!

The habit you want to target is (be specific): ______________________________

____

Your top-three reasons for making this habit change are:

1.

2.

3.

When you feel like giving up on your habit change, you want to remind yourself that (encouragements to get past a tough period):

1.

2.

3.

Your habit change team (people who will be supportive of your habit change and who would be there to help you get past a difficult period):

1.

2.

3.

Top cues for your habit:

Situational	Emotional
1.	1.
2.	2.
3.	3.
4.	4.

- ☐ Chew gum
- ☐ Use a squeeze ball
- ☐ Fiddle with a pencil
- ☐ Drink a glass of cold water
- ☐ Review your quit motivations
- ☐ Call a friend/team member
- ☐ Other:
- ☐ Other:

- ☐ Complete a breathing exercise
- ☐ Jog in place briefly (or do jumping jacks)
- ☐ Do 10 push-ups
- ☐ Engage with your smartphone
- ☐ Move out of a high-risk situation
- ☐ Other:
- ☐ Other:

Your quit date (the date you select for giving up your habit) is: ___________

Prior to your quit date you should:

- ☐ Inform your habit change team of your quit date.
- ☐ Feel really good about your plan to get control over a bad habit!

GOALS

- To add variety to your exercise routine
- To set new goals
- To make use of other resources (classes, competitions)
- To continue logging your exercise sessions
- To handle lapses in your exercise program
- To make exercise a way of life

OVERVIEW

Variety is the key to maintaining a strong exercise habit over time. Although you may stick with the exact same type of exercise over time, the way in which you do it, the features you pay attention to, and the goals that are meaningful to you are likely to change. This program encourages this process, and this chapter discusses some ways you can add variations to your exercise program to keep it fresh, interesting, and rewarding.

Variation: The Key to Long-Term Success

Many of the changes you may want to consider are subtle. Changing the music you listen to, or exchanging music for podcasts or audiobooks, can renew the fun you experience during exercise. For example, if exercise becomes a time to listen to music (maybe exploring to a new artist), then it becomes easier to look forward to and settle into the exercise time regardless of your interest in "working out." Likewise, changing where you exercise (trying a new gym, changing your running route, inviting along a new exercise partner) can be a powerful way to make sure that exercise time feels like quality time. In fact, as exercise becomes easier and more automatic, you may well find that you have a greater ability to supplement exercise with other features (the Exercise+ approach; attending to music, mindfulness, friends, or a new route) to make your exercise time feel much more like personal time. Moreover, if you are meeting the goal of working out four times a week, feel the freedom to make at least one of these weekly exercise sessions particularly special. For example, if you choose walking or running for your exercise, you may want to consider driving to a new location for your exercise (e.g., *It would be fun to run today through that cute town off Route 2*).

Setting New Goals

Another important feature of keeping exercise interesting over the longer term is allowing your goals for exercise to change. The primary aim for exercise, relative to this workbook, is to achieve mood benefits. Nonetheless, over time continued exercise will possibly lead to other changes, including weight loss and changes in the shape of your body. Paying attention to and enjoying these changes can motivate you in your long-term exercise program. However, you will want to make sure that these goals are appropriate to the *timeline* of change. For example, it takes a few months to change body shape. For this reason, you will not want to make changes in body shape a primary goal—it is just too hard to exercise only for this longer-term outcome. But if you are exercising because it helps you feel good *now*, then it is also appropriate to enjoy the longer-term changes in body shape. So, don't be in a hurry to achieve results, but do enjoy the body shape changes that occur.

If you are losing weight with exercise, it is because you have changed the basic equation necessary for weight loss—expending more calories than you are taking in. And, it is likely that you have done so in the preferred way—increasing the burning of calories with exercise rather than just restricting your eating. Also, with regular exercise and the mood benefits it brings, you may find yourself less interested in eating as a strategy for coping with feeling down, bored, or lethargic.

A number of body shape changes may be taking place as you exercise, independent of weight change. Certain muscles will become stronger, and as you continue to enjoy exercise, you may choose different body shape goals. For example, you may want to select exercises to reshape the chest and neck, the abdominals, or the hips or thighs. Personal trainers are experts at how to target these regions.

Use of Other Resources: Classes and Competition

Once your body begins to respond to exercise and you feel yourself getting in shape, you may want to consider other ways to increase or assess your fitness. You may want to think about joining classes or participating in fun competitions. Classes can extend the range of activities in which you can comfortably participate. They can also lead you a long way forward in developing a group of supportive co-exercisers. For competitive events, the key here is to focus only on those that you find enjoyable. In most cities, there is a wide variety of competitions available. For example, events for running range from charity walks or runs, fun runs (particularly on holidays), and community races, to serious competitions. In recent years, access to half-marathons, marathons, and triathlons has increased dramatically. For many of the casual participants in these events, the goal is to finish, or finish with a sense of competence, rather than to finish with a certain time in mind. These events are useful for honing your training efforts: There is something specific to practice and strive for in weekly exercises. They also provide a sense of group participation, a day of activity and celebration, and often a T-shirt or other reward for participating. The water stations along the way, and free water, fruit, or yogurt at the finish line, also add a nice level of drama and reward to the day of the race.

If you think any of these features would be useful to help you gain more joy from your exercise routine, check websites and running clubs in your area for information. Also, it is important to know that competitions can extend to a range of other activities, including gym-based competitions, swimming clubs (see masters' clubs on the web), sports clubs (softball, volleyball, basketball, pickleball, and hockey), and specialized competitions such as rock climbing.

As exercise becomes more of a habit, Worksheet 5.6: Exercise for Mood Log will lose some of its usefulness, and we have designed Worksheet 14.1: Monthly Exercise Log to help you keep a diary of the nature and quality of your exercise program. This updated worksheet offers you a way to target frequent exercise (averaging four days a week) and keep track of trends in your exercise, including exercise sessions you found particularly enjoyable. It also provides you with space for coaching yourself toward new exercise goals. This worksheet can be found at the end of this chapter or can be accessed by searching for this book's title on the Oxford Academic platform, at academic.oup.com. If you prefer to log your exercise sessions online instead of on paper, or if you are interested in logging other health habits (e.g., sleep or nutrition) as well, you may want to join a free service like MapMyRun (http://www.mapmyrun.com) or Fitlink (http://www.fitlink.com).

Handling Lapses in Your Exercise Program

As you exercise over the long term, you may also face the reality of lapses in your exercise habit. There may be times that you slip away from regular exercise, suddenly realizing that you have gone for a week or two with no organized activity. If this happens, you will need to be a good coach to yourself with the following steps:

1. Understand that such slips in motivation are natural.
2. Take some time to think what can be done to make your next exercise session especially enjoyable.
3. Remind yourself that you are exercising to feel good and/or to sharpen cognition.
4. Try to restart your exercise routine before you start to feel a change in your fitness level.

Keep in mind that going back to exercise when you are feeling fit, regardless of your level of motivation in the moment, is a much easier process than waiting for stronger motivation to return. Remember to exercise first and feel the motivation to exercise second.

As you continue to exercise, you will find yourself developing habits that further support your exercise goals. You may notice that you have a variety of workout clothes, and that you've perfected the process of where to hang sweaty clothes as they await their time in the washer. You may find yourself looking forward to the feeling of muscle heaviness or soreness that follows a particularly good exercise session. On trips, you may find that you use your walks or runs to get to know the new city, and that asking for a running route or information on the gym becomes part of your hotel check-in routine. If you find yourself starting these new habits, let yourself enjoy the degree to which you have made an exercise routine part of your life-balancing strategies and your mood-regulation efforts. Then go tell your friends about it.

Be sure to congratulate yourself on your accomplishments with this program thus far. Your feeling of success may further motivate you to keep exercising. But remember, you don't have to wait to feel motivated. Go ahead and use exercise to feel good *now*!

Worksheet 14.1: Monthly Exercise Log

Exercise session	Exercise completed	Duration and intensity	Notes and plans
1			
2			
3			
4			
5			
6			
7			
8			
9			
10			
11			
12			
13			
14			
15			
16			
Bonus			
Bonus			
Bonus			

Comments on the month: ____

Special goals or plans for the next month: _______________________________